HANDBOOK OF ICU THERAPY

HANDBOOK OF ICU THERAPY

Edited by
Ian McConachie
MBChB, FRCA

ISBN 1 900151 782

First Published 1999

Distributed worldwide by
Oxford University Press

Project Manager
Gavin Smith

Production and Design by
Saxon Graphics Limited, Derby

Printed in Great Britain by
Ashford Colour Press

PREFACE

This text:

- Is aimed primarily at trainees working in intensive care. Hopefully it will appeal to multidisciplinary trainees being exposed to ICU for the first time under joint college guidelines for ICU training. It may also be of interest to ICU nurses looking for information on modern medical (in the strictest sense) approaches to ICU therapy. A basic knowledge of physiology and pharmacology is assumed as well as either a medical background or advanced nursing experience in intensive care.
- May also be a useful *aide-mémoire* for ICU examinations especially for the FRCA and future diplomas in intensive care.
- Arose out of a series of ICU study days organized by the Editor in the North West region since 1992. All the authors have been lecturers on these courses. The other main source and inspiration for this text was a folder of 'Guidelines for Therapy' written by the author in 1991 and 1993 while working at a previous hospital.
- The authors are all either experienced ICU practitioners or invited experts on specialist issues. Being involved in ICU research was not a prerequisite although many of the authors have been or are involved in ICU research – a clinical commitment at the bedside was thought more important for this text.
- Aims to provide practical information on the management of common and/or important problems in the critically ill patient as well as sufficient background information to enable understanding of the principles and rationale behind their therapy. We hope it will prove useful at the bedside but we would like to emphasize that this, or any other book, is no substitute for experienced supervision, support and training.
- Emphasizes the importance of cardiac function throughout.
- Does not aim to cover all ICU practice and is not a substitute to the major ICU reference textbooks. For example, monitoring techniques

are not covered (best learnt at the bedside) but, however, the philosophy of monitoring is covered where necessary to illustrate important management points. Similarly, pathophysiology is included to help understand management principles.

- Has a format designed for easy access to information also presented in a concise manner. We have tried to eliminate all superfluous material. Selected important or controversial references are presented as well as suggestions for further reading.

Ian McConachie
Blackpool
June 1998

CONTENTS

Section II: Specific Problems

CONTRIBUTORS

Ian McConachie
MBChB, FRCA

Consultant in Anaesthesia and Intensive Care
Blackpool Victoria Hospital

Daniel R. Kelly
MBChB, FRCA

Consultant in Anaesthesia and Intensive Care
Blackpool Victoria Hospital

P. Nightingale
FRCA, MRCP

Consultant in Anaesthesia and Intensive Care
University Hospital of South Manchester

Nigel P.C. Randall
BM, FRCA

Consultant in Intensive Care Medicine and Anaesthesia
Blackpool Victoria Hospital

David Hesketh-Roberts
MD, FRCP

Consultant Cardiologist
Blackpool Victoria Hospital

Roop Kishen
MBBS, DA, MD, FRCA

Consultant in Intensive Care Medicine and Anaesthesia
Hope Hospital, Salford

C. Clarke
MB, ChB, FRCA

Consultant in Anaesthesia and Intensive Care
Blackpool Victoria Hospital

S.G. Brear
MBBS, FRCP

Consultant Physician
Wythenshawe Hospital, Manchester

CARDIAC FUNCTION, MONITORING AND OXYGEN TRANSPORT

CARDIAC FUNCTION, MONITORING AND OXYGEN TRANSPORT

Determinants of cardiac function

Heart rate and rhythm

Cardiac output (CO) = heart rate (HR) × stroke volume (SV).

- Therefore bradycardia will impair CO. Conversely, increases in HR, although arithmetically increasing CO, may impair overall cardiac function by increasing myocardial oxygen demand, causing ischaemia and reducing time for diastolic filling. Some units therefore use the response of SV to therapy as being more appropriate for overall cardiac function

- An arrhythmia may also be detrimental to cardiac function, e.g. in AF the loss of the atrial contribution to ventricular filling may be significant.

Preload

- The force of ventricular contraction is related to the myocardial fibre length (Frank Starling relationship).

- Myocardial fibre length is related to end diastolic ventricular volume (EDV). This is commonly referred to as 'preload'. The heart beats efficiently with adequate preload and thus fluid therapy may increase cardiac function.

- EDV is difficult to quantify though an assessment can be made by echocardiography.

- Vascular pressures can be measured more easily and both central venous pressure (CVP) and pulmonary artery occlusion or capillary 'wedge' pressure (PAOP or PCWP) are used clinically to reflect the end diastolic pressure (EDP) and thus the EDV.

- Graphs can be constructed of CO against filling pressure. Filling pressure can then be increased until there are no further increases in CO. Preload can then be considered to be optimal.

- One problem is that with decreased compliance (increased stiffness) of the ventricle wall, e.g. following myocardial infarction, the pressure may be increased relative to the volume. Therefore, the EDP may overestimate true preload.

Afterload

- Afterload is the force opposing contraction.

- There are several factors involved in afterload or impedance to ejection:

- Aortic diastolic pressure which the heart must overcome to eject blood.

- Peripheral resistance in the circulatory system. Clinically this is reflected by systemic vascular resistance (SVR). SVR = mean arterial pressure (MAP) – CVP/CO.

- Tension across left ventricle wall. This is dependant on the EDV, EDP and intrathoracic pressures (especially when these are increased during mechanical ventilation).

- Blood viscosity; increases in viscosity increase impedance to ejection and reduce flow.

Contractility

- The force and velocity of cardiac contraction is one definition of contractility although this is very difficult to measure in practice as most clinical measurements, e.g. CO, ejection fraction, etc. are influenced by preload and afterload.

- CO, stroke volume, left ventricular stroke work and ejection fraction are best thought of as measures of overall cardiac performance which is probably clinically more useful.

- Positive inotropic drugs increase contractility while ischaemia reduces contractility.

Echocardiography

Echocardiography, especially by the transoesophageal route, is a useful, comparatively non-invasive means of assessing cardiac function. Advantages include:

- dynamic as opposed to static assessment, e.g. one can see how the heart functions globally and see regional wall motion abnormalities;

- easy assessment of cardiac, valvular and major vessel structures;

- it helps provide the 'missing link' between pressure and volume within the cardiac chambers.

Limitations of CVP monitoring

- CVP reflects right atrial pressure, which is usually taken to reflect right ventricle (RV) end diastolic pressure.

- It does not necessarily reflect left ventricle (LV) preload and also poorly correlates with blood volume. CVP is often used as a guide to LV function and, indeed, directional changes in CVP may reflect alterations in LV performance. However, if either ventricle becomes selectively depressed, or in the presence of severe pulmonary disease, changes in CVP will not reflect changes in LV function.

- CVP is 'several steps' away from LVEDV or true preload and each approximation is influenced by pathological conditions, e.g. LV compliance, mitral valve disease, intrathoracic pressures, tricuspid regurgitation.

- There are many studies showing a poor relationship between CVP and PCWP in various disease states.

- CVP provides useful information regarding the status of the right side of the heart. This is valuable in cases of RV failure or in assessing the RV response to pulmonary hypertension.

Pulmonary artery flotation catheter (PAFC)

The pressure recorded when the pulmonary artery catheter is 'wedged' in a small branch of the pulmonary artery (the pulmonary capillary wedge pressure, or PCWP) is accepted as a close approximation of the left atrial (LA) pressure.

- Despite its limitations the PAFC is accepted as the best available indicator of preload and also allows measurement of cardiac function.

- Modern variants of the PAFC permit pacing, continuous cardiac output measurement, continuous display of mixed venous oxygen saturation (SVO_2) and RV ejection fraction measurements.

Indications

- Monitor preload and cardiac output.

- Optimize preload prior to the use of inotropes.

- Pulmonary oedema if is not responsive to simple measures or where therapy produces hypotension.

- Shock unresponsive to simple measures.

- Complicated myocardial infarction (MI).

- Differentiate cardiogenic and non-cardiogenic pulmonary oedema.

- May be inserted prophylactically for high risk surgery and cardiac surgery

Pitfalls in the PCWP

- Upper limit of 'normal' is 12 mmHg. The optimal PCWP is the one that provides the best CO without increases in lung water or pulmonary oedema. The optimal PCWP is rarely above 18 mmHg.

- It is only a guide to the LA pressure. Pulmonary artery (PA) diastolic pressure usually approximates to PCWP and may sometimes be used if there is difficulty getting the catheter to 'wedge'.

- If compliance is increased, e.g. after previous MI, it is accepted that PCWP will usually have to be greater than 'normal' for optimal stroke volume.

- Can reflect transmitted intrathoracic pressure, especially in the presence of positive end expiratory pressure (PEEP). To minimize the effect of intrathoracic pressure on PCWP the catheter tip should be positioned in the lower one-third of the lung (if higher, alveolar pressure may exceed pulmonary artery pressure). All PCWP measurements should be made at end of expiration (EE).

   During spontaneous respiration, EE = highest part of waveform.
   During IPPV, EE = lowest part of pressure waveform.

- Is not a measurement of blood volume although changes in PCWP correlate with changes in blood volume.

Thermodilution cardiac output and derived haemodynamic variables

- Thermodilution PAFC measures temperature in the PA (a useful source of an accurate core temperature). 10 ml of cold fluid is injected through the proximal port of the catheter. Blood flow is calculated from the temperature drop sensed by the Thermistor after mixing has occurred.

- The CO measured in this way is currently viewed as the 'Gold Standard' method of this measurement in the critically ill patient.

- CO varies with height and weight. To enable one patient to be compared with another the CO is usually indexed to body surface area (BSA) – the cardiac index (CI). In theory, every patient has the same 'normal' CI.

- Because of the differences in cardiac output with changes in intrathoracic pressure during IPPV, some recommend timing the measurement at end of expiration. However, this begs the question: which is the 'correct' CO; the one during inspiration or the one during expiration? It seems sensible to make the measurements randomly and to obtain an 'average' CO.

Derived haemodynamic variables

- Stroke work index (SWI) is the work generated by each ventricle during one cardiac cycle. It is a function of the pressure generated in systole and the SV ejected. Increases in SWI may be beneficial but also increases myocardial oxygen demand.

- Vascular resistance, systemic or pulmonary. Resistance is determined by dividing the pressure drop across the system by flow. There is controversy as to whether SVR and PVR should be indexed to BSA. The main use of the SVR is to help sort out the specific problem in cases of hypotension, especially in septic shock but one should treat the BP rather than the SVR. SVR may be increased by vasoconstriction or hypertension. Reductions occur in sepsis, cirrhosis and AV fistulae. Changes in calculated SVR may be seen with changes in CVP without any change in vascular tone.

Normal values

$$LVSWI = (MAP - PCWP) \times SVI \times 0.0136 \qquad 44\text{--}56 \text{ g.m/m}^2$$

$$RVSWI = (PAP - CVP) \times SVI \times 0.0136 \qquad 7\text{--}10 \text{ g.m/m}^2$$

$$SVR = \frac{MAP - CVP}{CO} \times 80 \qquad 900\text{--}1200 \text{ dynes.s/cm}^5$$

$$PVR = \frac{MPAP - PCWP}{CO} \times 80 \qquad 100\text{--}200 \text{ dynes.s/cm}^5$$

MPAP = mean pulmonary artery pressure.

The PAFC controversy

- Detractors of the PAFC state that their benefit in terms of increased survival is unproved. Of course, survival will not be improved by any monitoring or measurements. Survival will only be improved if appropriate therapeutic measures are taken on the basis of the measurements taken. The use of a PA catheter is only of value if used as part of an overall management plan.

- An important paper was published in 1996 and caused considerable discussion. It claimed to show an increased mortality associated from the use of the PAFC.[1] Direct complications, e.g. arrhythmias, pulmonary infarction, were not thought to be responsible as these are, in general, low in experienced hands. The increased mortality is thought to arise from inappropriate use of the information obtained especially inappropriate use of 'supranormal goals' of oxygen transport as discussed below. Although there is disagreement with the methodology of this study (e.g. it was retrospective) there are now calls for formal controlled studies of the use of the PAFC in critically ill patients (which might previously have been considered unethical).

- In addition, inappropriate use of the information obtained from the PAFC may be compounded by the ignorance of doctors inadequately trained in their use.[2]

However, there is no doubt that the PAFC gives us invaluable information, not readily obtained elsewhere. For example:

- In one study[3] physicians were only able to predict correctly values for PCWP, CI and PA pressure ~50 % of the time. Treatment was changed in 48.4% of patients after catheterization. This is not meant to suggest that all critically ill patients should have a PAFC since the most important role of the experienced physician is in deciding who should be catheterized, and when.

- A French study found correctly predicted haemodynamic profiles in only 56% of patients prior to catheterization. Changes of treatment were prompted in 63% of patients who were unresponsive to standard therapy. The mortality rate was significantly less when the assessment of haemodynamic data led to a change in therapy despite identical pre-catheterization characteristics.[4]

- Many other instances of the value of the PAFC will be found in other chapters of this text. Studies may help define the best therapies in differing circumstances. Improvements in survival may then be demonstrated.

Oxygen transport

Oxygen delivery, or DO_2, is the oxygen content of the arterial blood (CaO_2) multiplied by blood flow or CO.

Thus, $DO_2 = CO \times CaO_2$.

The normal CaO_2 of 20 ml is the haemoglobin (Hb) concentration multiplied by 1.34 (the constant for the amount of O_2 each g Hb can combine with) and the % oxyhaemoglobin saturation (SaO_2). Dissolved O_2 is usually considered negligible. This is the CaO_2 per decilitre which must, therefore, be multiplied by 10 to unify the units because CO is measured in l/min,

i.e. $DO_2 = CO \times Hb \times SaO_2 \times 1.34 \times 10$.

Normal DO_2 therefore

$5 \times 15 \times 100\% \times 1.34 \times 10 = \sim 1000$ ml/min.

If CI is used the resultant DO_2 is also indexed to BSA.

i.e. $DO_2 = \sim 600$ ml/min/m².

Adequate DO_2 is achieved by attention to cardiac function, Hb and oxygenation. Note that the PaO_2 contributes little to oxygen content and DO_2 (PaO_2 is not an important measure of arterial oxygenation. The SaO_2 is more significant in assessing oxygenation of arterial blood while the PaO_2 is important in evaluating gas exchange in the lungs).

Oxygen release from Hb at the tissues is increased by factors shifting the oxyhaemoglobin dissociation curve to the right, e.g. acidosis, fever, increased 2,3-DPG, while factors which shift the curve to the left, e.g. alkalosis, hypothermia, reduced 2,3-DPG (stored blood), impair oxygen release at the tissues.

In patients who are fully oxygenated and have an adequate Hb, the only logical way to increase DO_2 is to increase cardiac index. This has practical implications for therapy.

Normal mixed venous oxyhaemoglobin saturation (SVO_2) is 75% (68–77%) and therefore venous oxygen content (CvO_2) is 15 ml. Thus the oxygen extraction ratio (OER) is 25%. Oxygen consumption (VO_2) of the whole body (indexed) is therefore:

$VO_2 = CI \times (CaO_2 - CvO_2) \times 10 = \sim 150$ ml/min/m².

VO_2 reflects metabolic rate and as such is increased in thyrotoxicosis, fever, physiological stress response, feeding and by a direct calorigenic effect of inotropes.[5] Anaesthesia, cyanide and carbon monoxide poisoning, and hypothermia reduce VO_2. Sedation of ventilated patients reduces VO_2 partly by direct sedative effect and partly by reducing the work of breathing.

Supply dependency

- The normal response to a fall in DO_2 (low CI, anaemia, hypoxaemia) is to maintain VO_2 by increases in OER and decreases in SVO_2. Thus, normally, VO_2 is 'supply independent'.

- VO_2 is 'supply dependant' when extraction does not change in response to alterations in delivery, i.e. further increases in DO_2 result in increases in VO_2 – revealing potential tissue hypoxia. Supply dependency was widely identified in early studies where DO_2 and VO_2 were calculated using the shared variables of CI and CaO_2. This leads to a potential error due to 'mathematical coupling'. This finding led to many studies of increasing DO_2 to 'supranormal' levels which is generally no longer recommended.[6] More recent studies, using truly independent methods of measuring DO_2 and VO_2, have mainly failed to substantiate the claims for widespread existence of supply dependency.[7]

- In addition, if dobutamine has a direct calorigenic effect to raise VO_2,[5] then this response need not reflect tissue hypoxia.

- There are frequent 'spontaneous' changes in DO_2 and VO_2 in ventilated patients.[8] This limits the value of studies showing that VO_2 is dependent on DO_2.

- There are still areas of controversy, for example, if the studies showing supply dependency were due to mathematical coupling why did studies of some groups of patients show this (e.g. septic and ARDS patients) while other groups (e.g. heart failure) did not?

At the other end of the scale, with decreases of DO_2:

- Where DO_2 is low and lactic acidosis present, increasing DO_2 will lead to increases in VO_2,[9] i.e. supply dependency. In haemorrhagic or cardiogenic shock, VO_2 is maintained by increases in OER down to a critical level of DO_2 (below which further decreases in DO_2 lead to the rapid demise of the patient) at the expense of low levels of SVO_2.

- This mechanism of increased extraction is only a short-term answer and the O_2 debt has to be repaid. Studies have shown that the magnitude of O_2 debt and its clearance is linked to ultimate survival.[10]

Supranormal goals

- The team led by W.C. Shoemaker identified values of CI, DO_2 and VO_2 and blood volume retrospectively associated with increased survival of trauma and high risk surgical patients.[11] The 'goals' were:

- CI >4.5 l/min/m^2;

- DO$_2$ >600 ml/min/m^2;

- VO$_2$ >170 ml/min/m^2;

- normal BP; and

- blood volume 500 ml $>$normal unless PCWP >20 mmHg.

- They then attempted to achieve these goals prospectively in an attempt to improve survival in a similar group of patients with considerable success.[12]

- Others attempted to apply these goals in other groups of patients with lesser success.

- Indeed, it now seems that this approach may be detrimental in some groups of patients, e.g. the elderly in whom attempts to raise CI aggressively may promote myocardial ischaemia.[13]

- Thus it has been concluded that this approach cannot be universally recommended[6] but there may be benefits in specific groups of patients especially trauma patients and high risk surgical patients when applied preoperatively.

Monitoring of venous oxygenation

- SVO$_2$ can be measured by sampling blood from the pulmonary artery and measuring oxyhaemoglobin saturation via a co-oximeter or using an oximetric PAFC which continuously display the SVO$_2$.[14]

- If the critically ill patient is to survive DO$_2$ must be restored to such a level that VO$_2$ can be maintained without critically low levels of SVO$_2$. SVO$_2$ levels $<60\%$ are dangerous and levels of $<40\%$ are incompatible with long-term survival.

- SVO$_2$ is therefore obviously related to the balance of DO$_2$ and VO$_2$ or more accurately to the balance between the ability to extract oxygen and DO$_2$.

- SVO$_2$ does not necessarily vary with CO. Not all patients can increase their OER if DO$_2$ falls, e.g. septic patients with loss of vasoregulation and maldistribution of flow.

- Thus the value of mixed venous oxygenation measurements is that it reflects the balance between cardiac output and OER. As cardiac output is the most important index of DO$_2$ in most patients, many physicians monitor oxygen transport by measuring cardiac output and assessing its adequacy to metabolic needs with measurements of venous oxygenation.[15]

- The main flaw in this approach is that global measurements take little notice of regional disturbances.

Indices of tissue perfusion and oxygenation

Measurement of pHi (gastric mucosal pH) may be an indicator of splanchnic perfusion and may predict outcome.[16] Both pHi and blood lactate may be superior to oxygen transport variables in predicting outome.[17]

Further Reading

Pulmonary Artery Catheter Consensus Conference: Consensus Statement. *Crit Care Med* 1997; **25**: 910–25.

Shephard JN, Brecker SJ, Evans TW. Bedside assessment of myocardial performance in the critically ill. *Intensive Care Med* 1994; **20**: 513–21.

Poelaert J, Schmidt C, Colardyn F. Transoesophageal echocardiography in the critically ill. *Anaesthesia* 1998; **53**: 55–68.

Groeneveld AB, Kolkman JJ. Splanchnic tonometry: a review of physiology, methodology, and clinical applications. *J Crit Care* 1994; **9**: 198–210.

Soni N, Fawcett WJ, Halliday FC. Beyond the lung: oxygen delivery and tissue oxygenation. *Anaesthesia* 1993; **48**: 704–11.

References

1. Connors A, Speroff T, Dawson N *et al*. The effectiveness of right heart catheterisation in the initial care of critically ill patients. *JAMA* 1996; **276**: 889–97.

2. Gnaegi A, Feihl F, Perret C. Intensive care physicians' insufficient knowledge of right heart catheterisation at the bedside: time to act ? *Crit Care Med* 1997; **25**: 213–20.

3. Connors AF, McCaffree DR, Gray BA. Evaluation of right heart catheterisation in the critically ill patient without myocardial infarction. *N Engl J Med* 1983; **308**: 263–7.

4. Mimoz O, Rauss A, Rekik N *et al*. Pulmonary artery catheterization in critically ill patients: a prospective analysis of outcome changes associated with catheter-prompted changes in therapy. *Crit Care Med* 1994; **22**: 573–9.

5. Bhatt SB, Hutchinson RC, Tomlinson B *et al*. Effect of dobutamine on oxygen supply and uptake in healthy volunteers. *BJA* 1992; **69**: 298–303.

6. Heyland DK, Cook DJ, King D *et al*. Maximizing oxygen delivery in critically ill patients: a methodologic appraisal of the evidence. *Crit Care Med* 1996; **24**: 517–24.

7. Hanique G, Dugernier T, Laterre PF *et al*. Significance of pathologic oxygen supply dependency in critically ill patients: comparison between measured and calculated methods. *Int Care Med* 1994; **20**: 12–18.

8. Villar J, Slutsky AS, Hew E, Aberman A. Oxygen transport and oxygen consumption in critically ill patients. *Chest* 1990; **98**: 687–92.

9. Vincent JL, Roman A, De Backer D, Kahn RJ. Oxygen uptake/supply dependency. Effects of short-term dobutamine infusion. *Am Rev Resp Dis* 1990; **142**: 2–7.

10. Shoemaker WC, Appel PL, Kram HB. Role of oxygen debt in the development of organ failure sepsis, and death in high-risk surgical patients. *Chest* 1992; **102**: 208–15.

11. Shoemaker WC. Relation of oxygen transport patterns to the pathophysiology and therapy of shock states. *Int Care Med* 1987; **13**: 230–43.

12. Shoemaker WC, Appel PL, Kram HB *et al*. Prospective trial of supranormal values of survivors as therapeutic goals in high-risk surgical patients. *Chest* 1988; **94**: 1176–86.

13. Hayes MA, Timmins AC, Yau EH *et al*. Elevation of systemic oxygen delivery in the treatment of critically ill patients. *N Engl J Med* 1994; **330**: 1717–22.

14. Armaganidis A, Dhainaut JF, Billard JL *et al*. Accuracy assessment for three fiberoptic pulmonary artery catheters for SvO_2 monitoring. *Int Care Med* 1994; **20**: 484–8.

15. Vincent JL. The relationship between oxygen demand, oxygen uptake, and oxygen supply. *Int Care Med* 1990; **16 (suppl. 2)**: S145–8.

16. Doglio GR, Pusajo JF, Egurrola MA *et al*. Gastric mucosal pH as a prognostic index of mortality in critically ill patients. *Crit Care Med* 1991; **19**: 1037–40.

17. Friedman G, Berlot G, Kahn RJ, Vincent JL. Combined measurements of blood lactate concentrations and gastric intramucosal pH in patients with severe sepsis. *Crit Care Med* 1995; **23**: 1184–93.

2

SHOCK

Shock is a very imprecise term for a common, life-threatening condition.

A modern, acceptable definition of shock might be 'a clinical syndrome resulting from tissue dysfunction secondary to inadequate perfusion and oxygenation', i.e. inadequate DO_2 and VO_2. Note that hypotension is not part of this definition; shock and hypotension are commonly linked but not synonymous. One can be hypotensive without being shocked and one can be shocked without being hypotensive. Some authorities would insist that unless lactic acidosis is present (indicating tissue hypoxia) one cannot be said to be 'shocked'.

Signs of shock include:

- Clinical:
    - low BP, e.g. <90 mmHg or 60mmHg below a previous basal level;
    - oliguria <0.5 ml/kg/h;
    - pale, sweaty skin, cool peripheries;
    - rapid, thready pulse; and
    - reduced conscious level.
- O_2 transport – DO_2 and VO_2 reduced:
    - SVO_2 <50%;
    - lactic acidosis.

Studies have shown that VO_2 decreases before any changes in blood pressure, urine output, etc.

Four main types of shock have classically been described:

- hypovolaemic – often haemorrhagic in nature;

- cardiogenic;

- septic; and, less commonly,

- anaphylactic (see below).

In addition some recognize:

- traumatic – effect of tissue injury in addition to haemorrhage will be discussed in the appropriate section of this volume. For completeness, some describe:

- obstructive – a special form of cardiogenic shock due to failure of left ventricle (LV) filling due to cardiac tamponade, pneumothorax or venocaval obstruction; and

- spinal – not described in this text but the haemodynamic picture is mainly one of vasodilation.

Pathophysiology

Although it is common and in many ways appropriate to think of shock in haemodynamic terms (see below), shock is simultaneously a systemic and a cellular disease leading ultimately to:

- decreased ATP production;

- membrane dysfunction;

- cellular swelling; and

- cell death.

Once cellular swelling occurs, restoration of local tissue perfusion may not be possible leading to continuing secondary ischaemia. Damage to other organs such as the lungs results from leukocyte sequestration and deposition in the pulmonary capillaries leading to increased pulmonary shunting and increased capillary permeability from release of inflammatory mediators. The reticuloendothelial system function is depressed, which decreases clearance of toxic materials, e.g. endotoxin, foreign proteins, immune complexes and platelet aggregates.

Tissue trauma from trauma and surgery has additional effects:

- complement activation;

- coagulation cascade activation;

- cytokine release; and

- granulocyte activation leading to the production of oxygen free radicals and endothelium dysfunction.

During recovery from shock after successful resuscitation there will be an oxygen debt to be repaid. Studies have shown that failure to repay this debt is associated with ongoing tissue hypoxia and organ failure.[1]

Therapeutic approach to the shocked patient

Unfortunately, our knowledge of the pathophysiological cellular events in shock outweigh our ability to modify these events. Therapy is still largely 'macroscopic', i.e. restoration of tissue perfusion not 'microscopic'.

Airway, oxygenation and ventilation

The threshold for intubation and ventilation of shocked patients should be low:

- Patients are unlikely to be able to guard their own airway. Frank vomiting is uncommon but silent aspiration common.
- IPPV will reduce the work and oxygen consumption associated with breathing and hopefully ensure oxygenation.
- Severe shock will cause hypoxia in the absence of respiratory disease due to a reduction in pulmonary blood flow and low SVO_2.[2]
- Cardiac function may be supported (see Chapter 6).

Circulatory support

Including attention to:

- heart rate and rhythm;
- preload;
- contractility;
- afterload;
- coronary perfusion and cerebral perfusion pressures;
- haematocrit.

Simple haemodynamic patterns may help in diagnosis of the cause of shock and guide cardiovascular management although mixed pathology may coexist, e.g.:

- hypovolaemic shock – low PCWP, low CI, high SVR;
- cardiogenic shock – high PCWP, low CI, high SVR;
- septic shock – low PCWP, high CI, low SVR.

A fluid challenge is appropriate in virtually all patients unless obviously suffering from gross congestive cardiac failure.

Specific therapy according to cause: see appropriate chapters

Progressive or refractory shock

Even in young patients it has been shown that myocardial failure contributes to the shocked state if the shock is maintained, i.e. eventually all shock states will have a degree of cardiogenic aetiology. This is due to a combination of poor coronary perfusion, acidosis or possibly a depressant factor released from ischaemic tissue. This will proceed to so-called refractory shock where loss of capillary vasomotor control leads to reduced tissue blood flow, sludging in the microcirculation, and cellular hypoxia and death. It has also been suggested that refractory shock may partly have a septic component from bacterial or endotoxin translocation across the gut wall.

The 'Golden hour'

- The original concept of a 'Golden hour' or a critical therapeutic 'window' of opportunity was applied to shock following traumatic injury, but it probably applies to the outcome following shock due to any cause. Although generally accepted as a principle, it was originally based solely on animal studies backed up later by circumstantial patient evidence.

- In general, if the duration of shock >1 h, mortality increases progressively due to development of refractory shock or from the insidious development of organ failure. If shock is prolonged the patient is likely to die at a later stage from organ failures – even if the original 'shock' is subsequently reversed.

- Thus, speed is of extreme importance in resuscitating shocked patients.

- Therefore, it is common to initiate treatment empirically while the specific cause is being identified although common sense should tell one that the young man presenting with a large gastrointestinal bleed is suffering from haemorrhagic shock! The urgency of the situation may warrant the use of vasopressors to maintain coronary perfusion pressure while other therapies and diagnostic procedures are being instituted.

Anaphylactic shock

In anaphlactic shock the trigger stimulus causes release of histamine, serotonin, slow release substance, kinins and other vasoactive materials mainly from mast cells. These substances act primarily on smooth muscle leading to peripheral and airway oedema (stridor may not appear until 80% of the airway is obstructed), bronchospasm and vasodilatation and capillary leakage. Some of the mediators may also act directly on the myocardium. The two major causes of death are 'shock' – including cardiac depression and laryngeal oedema.

Management[3] includes:

- withdrawing the trigger stimulus, basic life support and CPR;

- laryngeal oedema may require intubation or cricothyrotomy or may settle with nebulized adrenaline in less severe reactions;

- i.v. fluids especially colloids should be administered to restore plasma volume.

A 1 mm layer of subcutaneous fluid over the whole body is equivalent to a loss of ~1.5 litres extracellular fluid.

- The agent of choice in severe reactions is adrenaline by incremental dosage as required. Infusions may be required after the initial treatment especially following reactions to agents with a long plasma half-life such as artificial colloids. In addition to its beneficial cardiac effects, it is a specific antidote as it blocks mediator release from mast cells. If the i.v. route is not immediately available, adrenaline may be administered down the tracheal tube.

- Steroids are usually administered but they take several hours to have an effect.

- Salbutamol may help for persistent bronchospasm but aminophylline should probably be avoided as there is an increased risk of serious arrhythymias when given in the presence of increased adrenaline blood levels.

- Antihistamines such as piriton are of little value in acute anaphylaxis as they do not reverse the effect of histamine already released and have no effect on the actions of mediators other than histamine. Logically, many authors contend that if antihistamines are desired to be given, H_1 and H_2 receptors must both be blocked for maximum therapeutic effect.

Further Reading

Britt LD, Weireter LJ Jr, Riblet J *et al*. Priorities in the management of profound shock. *Surg Clin North Am* 1996; **76**: 645–60.

Chernow B. New advances in the pharmacologic approach to circulatory shock. *J Clin Anesth* 1996; **8 (suppl.)**: 67S–69S.

Mouchawar A, Rosenthal M. A pathophysiological approach to the patient in shock. *Int Anesthesiol Clin* 1993; **31**: 1–20.

References

1. Shoemaker WC, Appel PL, Kram HB. Role of oxygen debt in the development of organ failure, sepsis and death in high risk surgical patients. *Chest* 1992; **102**: 208–15.

2. Westbrook JL, Sykes MK. Peroperative arterial hypoxaemia. The interaction between intrapulmonary shunt and cardiac output. *Anaesthesia* 1992; **47**: 307–10.

3. Fisher M. Treatment of acute anaphylaxis. *BMJ* 1995; **311**: 731–3.

3

OXYGEN THERAPY

D Kelly

Gas flow into the lung varies sinusoidally. The flow rate at its peak can vary enormously and can reach >100 l/min. However $\sim$50–60 l/min is more common. The flow rate depends on several factors such as:

- patient size;

- muscle power and endurance;

- disease state;

- presence or absence of airflow obstruction;

- compliance of lung.

Intratracheal oxygen concentrations will only stay constant if the total gas flow is high enough to meet the demands of the patient at all points of the inspiratory cycle. Environmental air will be entrained to make up the shortfall if the delivery system fails to deliver a high enough flow.

Very few oxygen delivery systems meet these requirements and consequently intratracheal oxygen concentrations can vary enormously:

- both between patients using the same device;

- within the same patient using the same device but under different circumstances.

Because the delivered flow rate is not high enough at some point during inspiration, air is entrained which dilutes the actual FiO_2 as table 3.1 illustrates:

Table 3.1 – O_2 concentrations prescribed compared with O_2 concentrations delivered to trachea.

Apparatus	% O_2 delivered	% in Trachea		
		quiet breathing	normal breathing	hyperventilation
Face mask with nebulizer at 10 l/min	44	39.5	32.7	26
	60	53.4	50.3	41
	100	62.7	52	42
Face mask with nebulizer at 15 l/min	44	41.1	34.2	29.1
	60	52.5	46.1	40.1
	100	68.1	54	50.2
Venturi mask at 4 l/min	24	23.1	22	21
	28	24.2	23	21.4
Venturi mask at 8 l/min	35	32.3	30	26.2
	40	36.4	33.1	29.4

Adapted with permission from Gibson RL, Comer PB, Beckham RW, McGraw CP. Actual tracheal oxygen concentrations with commonly used oxygen equipment. *Anesthesiology* 1976; **44**: 73.

Delivery devices

Nasal catheters

Can be single or double pronged. The single catheters are more recent and are better tolerated due to a foam collar around their distal end. Nasal catheters are better tolerated by patients and are more likely to be kept on. However, as can be seen from table 3.1, the intratracheal FiO_2 varies with gas flow rate and patients' inspiratory flows.

Low flow masks

Masks such as the Hudson rely on the entrainment of air around the mask and through holes in the mask to meet the patients demand for gas and, as explained earlier, this can vary enormously. The higher the inspiratory flow rate, the more air is entrained and the lower the inspired FiO_2.

Low flow masks with reservoirs

Adding a reservoir for oxygen to these masks diminishes the amount of air that needs to be entrained to match the inspired flow rates and consequently the FiO_2 is higher. Oxygen has to be supplied at a high enough rate to keep the reservoir bag inflated. If this is achieved then the FiO_2 can be as high as 85%.

High flow masks

These masks entrain air using the oxygen supply as a jet stream. The fast-moving gas imparts energy to the static gas, i.e air and some of this gas is dragged along with the faster stream. These masks were traditionally known as venturi masks although it is not strictly a venturi effect which entrains the air.[1] The oxygen concentration is preset if the oxygen flows to the mask are set correctly. These masks are more likely to provide a more reliable intratracheal oxygen concentration. However, if the inspiratory flow rates are high even these delivery systems will not meet the needs of the patient and the intratracheal FiO_2 will be lower than prescribed.

T pieces

These are connected to endotracheal or tracheostomy tubes and are supplied with humidified air and oxygen from a variable entrainment device. At the higher oxygen concentrations the total gas flow is much less and dilution of the inspired FiO_2 from the open end of the T piece can be considerable. This can be reduced by adding a length of tubing to this open end which will then act as a reservoir of oxygen enriched air.

CPAP

This refers to constant positive airway pressure. These systems aim to maintain the airway pressure positive relative to atmospheric pressure at all phases of the respiratory cycle. They do this by utilizing expiratory valves which raise the pressure and either high flow rates or a mixture of high flow rates and a pressurized reservoir to minimize the fluctuations in pressure during the respiratory cycle. The work of breathing is minimized by keeping the degree of pressure fluctuation to a minimum. To maintain the system pressure it is important to minimize leakage. Tight-fitting face masks are mandatory and avoiding pressure effects from these can be difficult. Because of the closed nature of these systems and high gas flows utilized the FiO_2 is a much more reliable predictor of intratracheal oxygen concentrations.

Benefits of CPAP

- A predictable FiO_2.

- An increase in FRC.

- A reduction in the work of breathing because the increase in lung volume moves the lung to a more favourable part of its pressure volume curve.

- A reduction in pulmonary vascular resistance secondary to the improvement in lung volume and relief of hypoxaemia.

Disadvantages of CPAP

- It increases mean intrathoracic pressure which reduces venous return to the heart.

- It requires a certain amount of technical expertise to assemble the circuit correctly.

- The high gas flows are difficult to humidify.

- The tight-fitting face masks are sometimes poorly tolerated and cause pressure effects.

Oxygen toxicity

Many patients are denied the oxygen they need for optimal organ function because of misplaced fears of oxygen toxicity. Because of the sigmoid shape of the oxygen dissociation curve a minimum haemoglobin saturation of 90% should be aimed for as this will ensure adequate blood oxygen content in most clinical circumstances. There are some drugs whose ability to cause alveolitis is enhanced by a high oxygen environment. Bleomycin is the best known but there are a number of reports implicating amiodarone in acute pulmonary toxicity when the lung is exposed to an increased FiO_2.[2] In these circumstances the inspired oxygen should be kept as low as possible. Oxygen toxicity is further discussed in Chapter 6.

Hypoxic drive

During an exacerbation of chronic obstructive pulmonary disease ventilatory drive can be four times normal.[3] Administering oxygen will reduce the drive but it does not return to normal and remains elevated.[4] The reduction in drive however will lead to a rise in the $PaCO_2$. If this is clinically significant then consideration should be given to some form of ventilatory support. A saturation of 90% should be aimed for. This will avoid most of the consequences of hypoxaemia without reducing the respiratory drive unduly. It should be borne in mind that a hypoxaemic arrest is much more damaging than a hypercapnic respiratory arrest.

Further Reading

Powell JF, Menon DK, Jones JG. The effects of hypoxaemia and recommendations for postoperative oxygen therapy. *Anaesthesia* 1996; **51**: 769–72.

Leach RM, Bateman NT. Acute oxygen therapy. *Br J Hosp Med* 1993; **49**: 637–44.

References

1. Scacci R. Air entrainment masks: jet mixing is how they work; the Bernoulli and Venturi principles are how they don't. *Respir Care* 1979; **24**: 928.

2. Donica SK, Paulsen AW, Simpson BR *et al*. Danger of amiodarone therapy and elevated oxygen concentrations in mice. *Am J Cardiol* 1996; **77**: 109–10.

3. Aubier M, Murciano D, Fournier M *et al*. Central respiratory drive in acute respiratory failure of patients with chronic obstructive pulmonary disease. *Am Rev Resp Dis* 1980; **122**: 191–9

4. Schmidt G, Hall J. Assessment and management of patients with C.O.P.D. in the emergent setting. *JAMA* 1989; **261**: 3444–453.

4

FLUID THERAPY IN ICU

- Maintenance of normal hydration and electrolyte composition is essential in ICU patients.

- 'Volume loading' is an important principle of cardiovascular management and is the cornerstone of management of surgical and trauma patients.

- Conversely, over hydration may compromise respiratory function and be a factor in poor outcome from ICU care.

- To understand the principles of fluid therapy one must be aware of which body fluid compartment one is wishing to maintain or resuscitate, e.g.:

- intracellular space – deficits mainly H_2O;

- interstitial space – deficits H_2O and electrolytes;

- intravascular space – deficits of plasma volume and/or red blood cells (RBC); and

- surgical and trauma patients may suffer losses of so called 'third space' fluids (called because it represents a third extracellular space) due to tissue fluid sequestration of interstitial fluid, i.e. H_2O and electrolytes.

Fluid therapy involves the use of:

Crystalloids

- H_2O with electrolytes approximating the composition and osmolality of plasma.

- Crystalloids redistribute through the extracellular fluids and, therefore, only ~20% of the volume administered will remain in the intravascular space.

- Hartmann's solution (compound Ringer's lactate) is closest in electrolyte composition with that of plasma and interstitial fluid. It has a pH 6.7.

- 0.9% Saline ('normal' saline) contains 150 mmol/l of both sodium and chloride, i.e. slightly increased Na but greatly increased Cl, cf. plasma and interstitial fluid. Excess use can be associated with hyperchloraemic acidosis and hypernatraemia. It has a pH 5.7.

- Dextrose 5%. No electrolytes, just dextrose and H_2O. Usually considered with the crystalloids but technically is not one because it contains no Na. It has a pH 4.5. Its osmolality is lower than the other common crystalloids. May be useful in the Na overloaded patient to replace H_2O but otherwise plays little role in ICU therapy. Dextrose 5% is *not* a resuscitation fluid.

Colloids

- H_2O, electrolytes and other particles (synthetic or natural) large enough to remain in the intravascular space for several hours.

- Albumin solutions are natural colloids and are discussed in detail below.

- Synthetic colloids are mainly starches or gelatin compounds.

Starches

The commonest is Hetastarch 6% (Hespan) with a clinical effect within the intravascular space of ~6 h. The starch particles are taken up by the reticuloendothelial system but long-term effects of their retention in the body are not known. Opinions differ regarding effects on coagulation – main effect is probably to promote a dilutional coagulopathy if large volumes are administered. Pentastarch 10% is another starch fluid with a lower molecular weight, cf. Hetastarch – more readily broken down by the kidney and excreted.

Gelatins

Relatively cheap and widely used. The clinical effect in the intravascular space lasts 3–4 h. Overuse should be limited by fear of excessive haemodilution which can reduce DO_2 after an initial rise.[1] Coagulation effects are from haemodilution only.

Dextrans

Dextrans contain polysaccharides. Some practitioners make use of their antithromboembolic and antisludging properties in situations where peripheral perfusion is compromised. Apart from this, they are not routinely used in ICU because they interfere with crossmatching and large volumes may cause a coagulopathy.

Blood products

RBC products

The optimal haemoglobin (Hb) concentration is a matter of debate – especially in critically ill patients.

- The triggers for RBC transfusion have been found to be arbitrary in ICU patients;[2] but:

- anaemia in ICU patients is associated with an increased risk of death and transfusion reduces this risk.[3]

Many believe that a Hb concentration ~10 g/dl, although somewhat arbitrarily chosen, is sensible representing a compromise between oxygen carriage and effects of viscosity on tissue blood flow.

Blood products

- Platelet and clotting factor transfusions should only be used where documented deficiencies are present.

- Routine use in haemorrhage is probably unnecessary in the absence of deficiencies.

- Even if deficiencies are present may still not be indicated in the absence of overt bleeding.

- Fresh frozen plasma should not be wasted by being used as a plasma volume expander.

RBC substitutes (see Further Reading)

The risks and problems of blood transfusion, e.g. infection, ABO incompatability, temperature changes, microaggregates, inefficient oxygen carriage of old blood, have prompted a search for effective blood substitutes – meaning fluids that carry oxygen.

- Solutions of Hb are being investigated as a RBC substitute which could act as a plasma volume expander with oxygen-carrying capability. This would not require cross matching and would, presumably, have a long shelf life. In early studies cell debris damaged the kidney. 'Stroma free' Hb solutions are being developed which are less toxic. If early success and enthusiasm is maintained, DNA technology may result in widespread availability of genetically engineered Hb.

- Perfluorocarbons are oxygen carrying fluorocarbon emulsions.[4] They only carry small quantities of oxygen but have the advantage of penetrating ischaemic tissues due to their small size and rheological properties. At this stage their routine use in ICU cannot be anticipated.

Small volume resuscitation

An initial bolus of 20 ml/kg is often recommended as the initial fluid volume in resuscitation. Small-volume resuscitation aims to achieve the same initial haemodynamic response with 4 ml/kg fluid with, of course, advantages in terms of time requirements for infusion and storage space required.

- Commonest fluid studied has been 7.5% saline – significantly hypertonic.

- Acts by many mechanisms including redistribution of interstitial fluid to the intravascular space and decreased cellular swelling and tissue oedema.

- ↑BP, CI, renal blood flow.

- Short-lived effect unless combined with colloid. Ultimately the interstitial fluid will have to be replaced.

- Main role has been in field resuscitation to 'buy time'.[5]

- Excessive use will lead to hypernatraemia.

- Because of the reduced tissue oedema, may be useful in head injuries.[6]

The crystalloid versus colloid debate

- There has been controversy over the best type of fluid for resuscitation, i.e. crystalloids or colloids. Part of the problem is the lack of studies showing a sufficiently clear superiority of one fluid type over another, sufficient to convert its opponents and without reasonable criticisms of study methodology. There are several problems with most of the available studies, e.g. different species, fluids, injuries, illnesses, complications studied.[7]

- It is not widely appreciated that many of the original US studies of crystalloids versus colloids in trauma patients were flawed. This was because most patients in both groups were given blood transfusions. In the USA patients are commonly given whole blood (as opposed to packed red cells in the UK), i.e. both groups received colloid from the whole blood, i.e. there was no such thing as a pure crystalloid group. Perhaps it is not surprising that few differences in outcome were detected.[8]

- However, in most studies there is probably a skewed distribution of severity of sickness with a large group of patients who will do all right whichever fluid is given and a smaller group of patients who will die regardless of which fluid is given. These patients may mask (statistically speaking) a group of patients in whom choice of fluid may be critical. This possibility has been seized upon by the colloid enthusiasts!

There are certain statements regarding the colloid/crystalloid controversy which can be made which are reasonably accepted by both groups:

- Crystalloids replace interstitial losses. Colloids are superior at replacing plasma volume deficits – more quickly and lasting longer – giving greater increases in CI and DO_2. Crystalloid administration may also produce such increases but approximately three times as much will be needed with consequent delays in achieving goals of resuscitation

- Crystalloids are cheap. Colloids are more expensive. Many centres in the USA use crystalloids almost exclusively. However, it has been pointed out that whole blood may be a significant source of colloid in studies purporting to use no colloid.

- In most situations, e.g. routine surgery, both potentially give excellent results if appropriate amounts are used.

- Many studies show similar effects on respiratory function. Overdose of either may produce respiratory failure.

- Overdose of crystalloids certainly cause dramatic peripheral oedema. The importance of this with regard to outcome is disputed.

- Anaemia is better tolerated than hypovolaemia.

- There is no doubt that the best replacement for major blood loss is blood.

Most reasonable people do not take extreme positions in the debate. In most situations close monitoring especially with regard to fluid overload is more important than absolute choice of fluid. However, many believe in the 'Golden hour' for resuscitation and that, therefore, speed of resuscitation is crucial. Therefore, when restoration of blood volume, cardiac output and tissue perfusion is urgent colloids are preferable to crystalloid.

Maintenance strategies

- Fluid intake comes from TPN, enteral nutrition, colloids, crystalloids and medications especially antibiotics. Thermodilution CO measurements at 10 ml fluid per measurement must not be forgotten.

- Losses come from urine, faeces especially diarrhoea, skin and lung evaporation (increases in fever), haemorrhage, third space losses, N/G drainage and fistulae. Vascular fluid may be lost to the circulation in ICU patients due to increased capillary endothelium permeability ('leaky capillaries'). Humidified gases reduce the insensible lung H_2O losses in ventilated patients.

- Hormonal changes promote Na and H_2O retention following surgery.

- Less well appreciated is that some drugs promote fluid retention – notably steroids.

- During critical illness many patients' weight increases, probably reflecting increased endothelial permeability rather than excessive administration of fluids. This is associated with a poor outcome.[9] Whether removing or preventing this extra fluid which has accumulated as oedema fluid can improve this reduced outcome back to 'normal' is less certain. Certainly, the balance of opinion is shifting towards 'keeping the patient dry' (as long as organ perfusion is well maintained).[10]

Thus it is important to watch intake closely and match to output where possible. Useful points are:

- weighing the patient daily is important;

- minimize fluids required to administer medications;

- once patient is established on nutritional support may not require 'routine' maintenance crystalloids;

- dramatic weight gain should be resisted if necessary by the judicious use of low dose diuretics if haemodynamically tolerated; and

- abnormal surgical losses, e.g. from fistulae, diarrhoea, should be replaced with crystalloids.

Volume-loading strategies

- Hypovolaemia must be treated promptly to restore organ perfusion.

- The consequences of hypovolaemia are arguably more difficult to treat and carry a higher mortality than the consequences of over hydration.

- A volume challenge, e.g. 5 ml/kg colloid, is probably indicated in all cases of acute haemodynamic compromise.

- Inotropes can have disastrous consequences in the presence of hypovolaemia (see Chapter 8).

- Fluid administration with, e.g. colloid, is best guided by a response of increasing stroke volume (SV) as a result of increasing PCWP, i.e. stop administering colloid when there is no further increase in SV with more fluid.

- In the absence of a PAFC, CVP trends can be useful (the absolute CVP is not always that helpful in ventilated patients), e.g.:

  - no ↑CVP and BP with fluid → give more fluid;

  - ↑CVP and BP and then ↓ → give more fluid;

  - ↑CVP but no ↑BP then → no more fluid; and

  - ↑CVP but ↓BP then → no more fluid.

- Obviously overloaded, oedematous patients may still need colloid boluses to maintain CO and filling pressures, i.e. the intravascular volume may still be low. The use of vasopressors to maintain filling pressures in such patients is controversial as splanchnic vasoconstriction may occur.

- Although difficult to prove many specialists believe that colloids are better than crystalloids in oedematous patients with 'leaky capillaries', if only because less volume will probably need to be given and, therefore, be available to 'leak out'.

- Short, large-bore cannula give best flows for rapid volume loading.

The vexed question of albumin

The use of albumin solutions in ICU is controversial, relates to both fluid therapy and nutritional support and merits discussion in some detail.

- Until relatively recently albumin solutions were the only readily available colloid solution available in the USA.

- Albumin solutions are still relatively expensive and scarce in many areas. One US study had difficulty with patient inclusion due to an actual shortage of albumin.

- In ICU patients, albumin synthesis is reasonably well maintained but the vascular permeability to albumin increases and the effective volume of distribution is dramatically increased. In addition, albumin metabolism is also increased. Thus, albumin blood levels fall rapidly in critical illness and reflect the severity of illness and mortality rather than nutritional status.[11] Trends in albumin levels predict the difficulty of weaning from mechanical ventilation.[12]

- Albumin levels are relatively insensitive to nutritional support.

- Albumin blood levels improve as the underlying condition resolves, often accompanied by a spontaneous diuresis.

Proponents of the use of albumin justify its use by citing:

- Increases in colloid oncotic pressure (COP).

- Free radical scavenging, binding of drugs and toxic substances.[13]

- Increased incidence of diarrhoea in hypoalbuminaemia.

- Albumin is a 'natural colloid'.

- If it is appropriate to replace low levels of, e.g. Hb, electrolytes, etc., why not albumin?

However, the COP gradient is relatively well maintained and, thus, numerous studies have failed to find a relationship between low albumin levels and pulmonary oedema. Most studies, most recently by Rubin *et al.*,[14] have failed to find benefits from albumin supplementation in terms of length of stay, outcome, etc. despite significant increases in albumin levels. The only significant increase in the albumin group in all studies has been in costs!

Further reading

Dietz NM, Joyner MJ, Warner MA. Blood substitutes: fluids, drugs, or miracle solutions? *Anesth Analg* 1996; **82**: 390–405.

Traylor RJ, Pearl RG. Crystalloid versus colloid: all colloids are not created equal. *Anesth Analg* 1996; **83**: 209–12.

Griffel MI, Kaufman BS. Pharmacology of colloids and crystalloids. *Crit Care Clin* 1992; **8**: 235–53.

Shires GT, Barber AE, Illner HP. Current status of resuscitation: solutions including hypertonic saline. *Adv Surg* 1995; **28**: 133–70.

Soni N. Wonderful albumin? *BMJ* 1995; **310**: 887–8.

References

1. Beards SC, Watt T, Edwards JD *et al.* Comparison of the hemodynamic and oxygen transport responses to modified fluid gelatin and hetastarch in critically ill patients: a prospective, randomized trial. *Crit Care Med* 1994; **22**: 600–5.

2. Corwin HL, Parsonnet KC, Gettinger A. RBC transfusion in the ICU. Is there a reason? *Chest* 1995; **108**: 767–71.

3. Hebert PC, Wells G, Tweedale M *et al.* Does transfusion practice affect mortality in critically ill patients? *Am J Respir* 1997; **155**: 1618–23.

4. Faithfull NS. Fluorocarbons. Current status and future applications. *Anaesthesia* 1987; **42**: 234–42.

5. Mattox KL, Maningas PA, Moore EE *et al.* Prehospital hypertonic saline/dextran infusion for post-traumatic hypotension. The USA Multicenter Trial. *Ann Surg* 1991; **213**: 482–91.

6. Vassar MJ, Perry CA, Gannaway WL, Holcroft JW. 7.5% sodium chloride/dextran for resuscitation of trauma patients undergoing helicopter transport. *Arch Surg* 1991; **126**: 1065–72.

7. Gammage G. Crystalloid versus colloid: is colloid worth the cost? *Int Anesthesiol Clin* 1987; **25**: 37–60.

8. Velanovich V. Crystalloid versus colloid fluid resuscitation: a meta-analysis of mortality. *Surgery* 1989; **105**: 65–71.

9. Lowell JA, Schifferdecker C, Driscoll DF *et al.* Postoperative fluid overload: not a benign problem. *Crit Care Med* 1990; **18**: 728–33.

10. Schuster DP. Fluid management in ARDS: 'keep them dry' or does it matter? *Int Care Med* 1995; **21**: 101–3.

11. McCluskey A, Thomas AN, Bowles BJ, Kishen R. The prognostic value of serial measurements of serum albumin concentrations in patients admitted to an intensive care unit. *Anaesthesia* 1996; **51**: 724–7.

12. Sapijaszko MJ, Brant R, Sandham D, Berthiaume Y. Non-respiratory predictor of mechanical ventilation dependency in intensive care unit patients. *Crit Care Med* 1996; **24**: 601–7.

13. Emerson TE Jr. Unique features of albumin: a brief review. *Crit Care Med* 1989; **17**: 690–4.

14. Rubin H, Carlson S, DeMeo M *et al.* Randomized, double blind study of intravenous human albumin in hypoalbuminaemic patients receiving total parenteral nutrition. *Crit Care Med* 1997; **25**: 249–52.

5

NUTRITION

Nutrition is extremely important in the critically ill patient. In its absence there will be:

- muscle atrophy and weakness;
- decrease in immune function;
- decrease in wound healing;
- impaired weaning off IPPV;
- gut mucosal atrophy (still occurs with parenteral nutrition).

In the critically ill patient who is markedly catabolic the above may occur in a few days. Nutritional support improves nutritional status but there is little concrete evidence for a beneficial effect on survival. However, promoting ongoing malnourishment must be detrimental to the patient. Certainly >10,000 kcal cumulative caloric balance is associated with a poor outcome in ICU patients.[1] There is little evidence that nutritional support can reverse the negative nitrogen balance or catabolism which occurs in the critically ill patient. In which case the purpose of support is to *minimize* the negative nitrogen balance.

In simple, i.e. non-physiologically stressed, starvation the energy requirements in the first week are chiefly met by amino acids produced by protein breakdown forming glucose via gluconeogenesis. The body adapts to a protein-sparing metabolism in starvation but these changes are absent or opposed in the ICU patient. In addition:

- Sepsis results in a preferential metabolism of fat rather than glucose partly due to inhibition of the enzyme complex pyruvate dehydrogenase.

- Protein synthesis is increased for the inflammatory response, wound healing, acute phase proteins but protein breakdown is accelerated leading to a net negative nitrogen balance – the acute catabolic state.

- The hormonal stress response, catecholamines and cytokines especially tumour necrosis factor (TNF), are responsible for the changes compared with starvation.

- Reversal of these obligatory catabolic changes is not possible during severe physiological stress[2] – only reversed when the cause of the hormonal release is removed, i.e. resolution of the underlying condition. Gluconeogenesis cannot be inhibited completely by provision of adequate substrate in severe catabolism.[3]

- The muscle wasting from the catabolic changes is compounded by the prolonged immobilization which accompanies critical illness.

- 'Overfeeding'[4] will not promote a positive nitrogen balance until the underlying condition resolves *and* the patient is mobilizing. Body weight may increase but this is mainly fat and total body protein still falls.

- Growth hormone administration to stimulate a positive nitrogen balance seemed promising in early studies but later studies were stopped due to an excess mortality in study group.

- When the patient is recovering and mobilizing they are often discharged from the ICU. Energy and protein intake should be increased to allow weight gain.

Assessment of nutritional status

Malnutrition is very common in hospital patients

- Common sense clinical examination will be helpful, e.g. history of weight loss and food intake, measured versus usual weight, specific features, e.g. of vitamin deficiencies and signs of muscle weakness and atrophy. Measured height and weight should be compared to standard tables.

- Anthropometric measurements, e.g. triceps skin fold thickness and mid-arm muscle circumference, are crude, occasionally useful but are operator dependent to some degree and may not be reproducible.

- Blood tests:

  - Albumin as an index of visceral protein mass is useful in pure malnutrition. However, in ICU, influences of decreased synthesis due to liver disturbances and loss due to capillary leak confuse the picture (see chapter on fluid therapy).

  - Serum transferrin has been suggested as a better index of body proteins as it has a longer circulating half life and is not an acute phase protein.

- Lymphocyte count and skin tests for common allergens (an index of immune competence which is depressed in malnutrition) are useful in pure malnutrition but, again, are less useful in ICU.

- Of experimental interest at present are accurate measurements from bioelectrical impedance which quantitatively measures lean body mass.

In summary, there are no simple tests appropriate for assessing acute malnutrition in critically ill patients. Clinical impression and serial estimations of weight compared with premorbid weight are probably as useful as more complex tests.[5]

Reasons for feeding the critically ill patient

- To minimize the net negative balance and breakdown of the body's tissues.

- To provide precursors for the immune response, wound repair and hepatic protein synthesis.

- Provision of nutritional support may increase the protein synthesis rate even if it does not decrease the catabolic rate.

- Glucose administration is partly protein sparing[6] but this effect is blunted by sepsis.

- Even low rates of enteral feeding limit gut mucosal atrophy.

Timing of initiation of feeding

- Although many patients may seem to tolerate a short period of low or no caloric intake, the greater the degree of catabolism, the less the period of hypocaloric intake should be.

- Enteral nutrition (EN)should be attempted within 24 h if there are no contraindications due to the rapid onset of gut mucosal atrophy.

- If EN is not possible, total parenteral nutrition (TPN) should be commenced as soon as the patient is haemodynamically stable.

Energy and protein requirements

Formulae, e.g. Harris Benedict *estimate* the basal energy expenditure (BEE) based on the patient's age, weight and sex. Studies have shown that the mean metabolic rate (and therefore caloric requirement) approximates to BEE +30%. Adjustments are often made as percentage increases based on the degree of 'stress' and activity.[7] For clinical purposes 25–30 kcal/kg/day with the higher value for the 'most stressed patients', e.g. multiple injuries and major burns, is sufficient. When calculating requirements, an admission 'dry weight' should be used as most ICU patients gain weight (metabolically inactive oedema fluid) during their illness.

Protein losses can be measured but in practise 1–1.5 g/kg/day are required. Alternatively, protein intake can be assessed on the basis of a ratio of 150:1 of non-protein calories to nitrogen (~6 g protein = 1g nitrogen).

Indirect calorimetry *measures* energy expenditure based on measurements of oxygen consumption and CO_2 production. This may be useful as a research tool but:

- Errors, e.g. from leaks, are a problem especially when the patient is on a high inspired O_2 concentration.

- Once-a-day 'spot check' measurements may be inappropriately extrapolated to the whole 24 hour day.

- Measurements in some patients vary markedly from day to day.

- Marked differences have been reported from different studies of similar groups of patients. One review[8] concluded 'At present indirect calorimetry may be better viewed as an investigative tool than a necessary part of routine patient care'.

Composition of non-protein calories

There is still controversy over the ratio of fat-to-carbohydrate (CHO) intake in the critically ill patient.

Pro fat

- Lipid preferentially metabolized in sepsis especially medium chain fatty acids (MCFA).

- Lipid is a non-irritant to veins and theoretically can be given via a peripheral vein.

- Fat gives more calories per g compared with glucose (9 compared with 4).

- Requirement for essential fatty acids.

Con fat

- Lipid particles may be taken up by the reticuloendothelial system.

- Long chain fatty acid (LCFA) metabolism impaired in sepsis (due to a deficit of intracellular carnitine).

- Fat possesses little or no protein sparing effect.

- Hyperlipidaemia may impair oxygenation but changes are small and probably of little clinical significance.

Pro CHO

- Some protein-sparing effect especially if lipid is also given.

- Some glucose intake probably essential.

Con CHO

- Hyperglycaemia (see below).

- Limit to utilization – maximum uptake 4–6 mg/kg/min.

- Excess CHO leads to hepatic steatosis.

- Caution in respiratory failure (see below).

Most authorities recommend ~50% of non-protein calories be administered as fat. Note: if propofol is infused for sedation one must remember that this is dissolved in a fat emulsion equivalent to 10% intralipid.

Other nutritional requirements

- H_2O and standard electrolytes need to be supplied. Magnesium and phosphate supplements may be required.

- Vitamins, both fat and H_2O soluble should be supplied in the form of a commercial multivitamin preparation. Requirements are mainly not known with certainty in the critically ill patient and are often extrapolated from normal requirements. Water-soluble vitamins should be administered every day. Fat soluble vitamins are required at least twice a week. In the long-term, vitamins B12, K and folate supplements may be required. Currently there is great interest in the role of vitamins C and E as antioxidants.

- Specific elemental requirements, e.g. zinc and manganese, may also be supplied commercially. Trace elements with lesser or unknown requirements can be assumed to be supplied as contaminants of other fluids and in blood transfusions.[9]

- Commercially produced EN preparations are generally balanced nutritional sources.

Hyperglycaemia

- Common in the critically ill patient – hormonal changes and insulin resistance. May be related more to increased production from gluconeogenesis rather than decreased utilization (unless septic).

- Assess whether intake is too high prior to prescribing insulin.

- Accept blood sugar up to 10 mmol/l as 'normal' to avoid risk of hypoglycaemia with very 'tight' insulin regimens.

- Higher levels should *not* be viewed as innocuous. Associated with osmotic diuresis and increased infections.

Nutrition in respiratory failure

Malnutrition impairs respiratory muscle strength. On the other hand, glucose and amino acid infusions increase VO_2. Glucose oxidation produces more CO_2 per g than fat and, therefore, excess supply of glucose may increase CO_2 production, work of breathing and impair ability to be weaned from mechanical ventilation. Enteral feeds with an increased proportion of fat to carbohydrate may reduce CO_2 production and allow easier weaning[10] although this is still controversial. It is possible that avoiding excess calories may be as important in this matter as the source of the calories.

Novel nutritional substrates

In the past 10 years there have been three major trends in ICU nutrition:

- A shift from enteral to parenteral nutrition.

- A decrease in the total quantity of calories administered.

- An improvement in the *quality* of nutrients administered, i.e. novel substrates.

It should be emphasized that in many instances the administration of these novel substrates is supported by, at best, circumstantial evidence. Few are supported by adequate controlled studies. A recent editorial reminds us to ensure that sufficient amounts of 'conventional' nutrients are supplied before becoming over concerned with novel substrates.[11]

Medium chain fatty acids (MCFA) versus long chain fatty acids (LCFA)

(refers to the position of the first double bond in the carbon chain – LCFA usually ω6, MCFA usually ω3 – 'fish oils').

LCFA may affect the immune system as it can enter arachidonic acid pathways, e.g. forming prostaglandins, platelet-activating factor, leukotrienes. MCFA are utilized solely for energy and are not metabolized to active products. MCFA in some studies may have beneficial effects on protein balance and may have no effect on lung function.

Branched chain amino acids (BCAA)

BCAA (leucine, isoleucine and valine) are metabolized in skeletal muscle and, in theory, should decrease muscle protein breakdown if preferentially administered. In the body their main role may be to generate glutamine and alanine. Routine use at present is unsubstantiated.

Glutamine

- Not an essential amino acid, i.e. the body should be able to synthesize sufficient glutamine from other essential amino acids (however, it is considered important enough to be added to cell and tissue cultures in the biology laboratory).

- Despite this, it has been suggested that the synthesis of glutamine is inadequate in critical illness, i.e. a *conditional* essential amino acid.

- The role of BCAA to provide glutamine has led to interest in administering glutamine.

- An essential fuel for bowel mucosal cells (may protect bowel mucosa) and for fibroblasts, lymphocytes and macrophages.

- Forms ~50% of the body's amino acid pool.

- Plasma and muscle glutamine levels fall after burns, trauma and major surgery.[12]

- Not included in standard formulations of TPN as is relatively unstable in solution (also 'non-essential').

- Can be supplied via enteral supplements.

Arguably, of all the novel supplements, glutamine is supported by the strongest evidence of worth. Supplementation has been shown to lessen the negative nitrogen balance after injury and major surgery.[13] A recent study in a heterogeneous group of ICU patients found a significant improvement in outcome in those patients who received glutamine supplements.[14]

Arginine

Technically another non-essential amino acid but important for wound healing, collagen deposition and immune function.

OKGA (ornithine salt of ketoglutaric acid)

It was suggested that ketoacids of BCAAs could provide the carbon skeleton of essential amino acids by transamination without the penalty of excessive N_2 load.

Thus, it was suggested that OKGA could reduce the negative nitrogen balance in critical illness by 'recycling' amino acid nitrogen.

Nucleotides

- May stimulate the immune system.
- Absent in standard TPN.

Immunonutrition

The concept of certain nutrients, e.g. ω3 MCFA, nucleotides, arginine, directly stimulating the immune system in critically ill patients and therefore reducing infectious complications and improving outcome is extremely exciting.

- One study compared a standard enteral feed with a preparation (Impact®, Sandoz nutrition) containing the so-called immunonutrients found a reduced length of stay on average and a decrease in infectious complications in the immunonutrient group.[15]

- The same immune stimulating feed has been shown to improve various indices of immune status in ICU patients.[16]

- A more recent study of major gastrointestinal (GI) surgery found a reduced incidence of late complications in the study group with the same preparation.[17] Analysis showed substantial savings in the Impact group because of the reduced complications despite the greater comparative cost of this preparation.

Total parenteral nutrition (TPN)

- Only indicated if unable to feed the patient via the enteral route.
- More expensive.
- More metabolic problems.
- TPN associated with a reduced survival due to infectious complications in cancer patients receiving chemotherapy.[18]
- Requires dedicated central venous access (with all its complications).
- Incidence of infectious complications related to the care of the site rather than the type of site, e.g. tunnelled versus non-tunnelled.
- Usually administered as a 2.5- or 3-litre 'big bag' feed with all the nutritional components mixed in pharmacy in a laminar flow cabinet under strict aseptic conditions.

Enteral nutrition

- Eating is normal. The gut is not meant to be rested. Mucosal atrophy is rapid.

- Requires a functioning GI tract. Bowel sounds not essential for absorption. Gastric atony can be more of a problem but the tube can be placed distal to the stomach.

- Absorption/transit increased by cisapride.[19] Oral erythromycin also stimulates gut activity.

- Supports normal gut flora.

- Possibly reduces GI bleeding from stress ulcers.

- Decreases infectious complications in surgical patients.[20]

- May preserve the gut barrier and prevent bacterial or endotoxin translocation.

- Reduced incidence of acalculous cholecystitis.

- Many commercial preparations. All ~1 kcal/ml.

- Cheaper than TPN and with less metabolic and infectious complications.

- Elemental, i.e. predigested feeds only necessary in patients with short bowel syndrome following small bowel resection. High osmolarity may promote diarrhoea.

- No need for 'starter' diluted feeds. If problems occur, start at lower rate rather than diluting the feed.

- A 4 hour rest during the night is often recommended. Stomach acidity during this period may limit bacterial growth in the stomach.

- Continuous pump feeding better than intermittent bolus feeding – less risk of aspiration.

There is uncertainty from animal studies as to whether enteral feeding promotes a better outcome or whether TPN promotes a worse outcome due to higher rates of complications.

Routes

- 'Sip feeds' insufficient in critically ill.

- Short-term: nasogastric tubes and fine bore tubes – stomach, duodenum or jejunum either spontaneously or endoscopically.

- Long-term: oesohagostomy, gastrostomy, duodenostomy and jejunostomy – surgically introduced or percutaneously.

Fine-bore tubes are difficult to aspirate from, block easily and have few advantages in the critically ill patient.

Complications

- Aspiration – watch for large residual volumes.

- Infection/contamination – feeds are excellent bacteria growth media.

- Blockage of tubes – flush all medications with H_2O.

- Malposition of tubes – check with chest X-ray.

- Constipation – often due to inadequate H_2O intake or possibly lack of fibre.

- Diarrhoea. Very common; check for antibiotics and other medications as causes of diarrhoea. *C. difficile* infection must always be excluded. In the absence of these causes treat symptomatically rather than automatically stopping the feed. Fibre may be important.

Fibre

- Many believe that fibre should be added routinely as part of an enteral feed regimen. Short-chain fatty acids produced by its breakdown by gut bacteria are essential nutrients for the colon. It may support normal gut flora, bind bile salts, absorb water, reduce Gram-negative bacteria overgrowth and improve glucose intolerance.

- Reduces enteral feeding associated diarrhoea in non-critically ill patients but there are no studies showing definite benefit in ICU patients.[21]

Further Reading

Cerra FB, Benitez MR, Blackburn GL *et al*. Applied nutrition in ICU patients. A consensus statement of the American College of Chest Physicians. *Chest* 1997; **111**: 769–78.

Heyland DK, Cook DJ, Guyatt GH. Enteral nutrition in the critically ill patient: a critical review of the evidence. *Int Care Med* 1993; **19**: 435–42.

American Society for Parenteral and Enteral Nutrition Board of Directors. Guidelines for the use of parenteral and enteral nutrition in adult and pediatric patients. *JPEN* 1993; **14**: 15A–25A.

References

1. Bartlett RH, Allyn PA, Medley T. Nutritional therapy based on positive caloric balance in burn patients. *Arch Surg* 1977; **112**: 974–80.

2. Long CL, Schiller WR, Geiger JW. Gluconeogenic response during glucose infusions in patients following skeletal trauma or sepsis. *JPEN* 1978; **22**: 619–25.

3. Elwyn DH, Kinney JM Jeevanandam M. Influence of increasing carbohydrate intake on glucose kinetics in injured patients. *Ann Surg* 1977; **190**: 170–5.

4. Streat SJ, Beddoe AH, Hill GH. Aggressive nutritional support does not prevent protein loss despite fat gain in septic intensive care patients. *J Trauma* 1987; **27**: 262–6.

5. Baker JP, Detsky AS, Wesson DE. Nutritional assessment: a comparison of clinical judgement and objective measurement. *N Engl J Med* 1982; **306**: 969–72.

6. Long JM, Wilmore DW, Mason AD. Effect of carbohydrate and fat intake on nitrogen excretion during total intravenous feeding. *Ann Surg* 1977; **185**: 417–22.

7. Schofield WN. Predicting basal metabolic rate, new standards and review of previous work. *Human Nutrition: Clinical Nutrition* 1985; **39C (suppl. 1.5)**; 41.

8. Christman JW, McCain RW. A sensible approach to the nutritional support of mechanically ventilated critically ill patients. *Int Care Med* 1993; **19**: 129–36.

9. Berger MM, Cavadini C. Unrecognised intake of trace elements in polytraumatised and burnt patients. *Annales Françaises d'Anesthesie et de reanimation* 1994; **13**: 289–96.

10. Al-Saady NM, Blackmore CM, Bennett ED. High fat, low carbohydrate, enteral feeding lowers $PaCO_2$ and reduces the period of ventilation in artificially ventilated patients. *Int Care Med* 1989; **15**: 290–5.

11. Griffiths RD. Feeding the critically ill – should we do better? *Int Care Med* 1997; **23**: 246–7.

12. Askanazi J Carpentier YA, Michelsen CB. Muscle and plasma amino acids following injury; influence of intercurrent infection. *Ann Surg* 1980; **192**: 78–82.

13. Stehle P, Zanders J, Mertes N *et al*. Effect of parenteral glutamine peptide supplements on muscle glutamine loss and nitrogen balance after major surgery. *Lancet* 1989; **i**: 231–3.

14. Griffiths RD, Jones C, Palmer TEA. Six-month outcome of critically ill patients given glutamine supplemented parenteral nutrition. *Nutrition* 1997; **13**: 295–302.

15. Bower RH, Cerra F, Bershadsky B *et al*. Early enteral administration of a formula (Impact®) supplemented with arginine, nucleotides and fish oil in intensive care patients; Results of a multicentre, prospective, randomised clinical trial. *Crit Care Med* 1995; **23**: 436–49.

16. Kemen K, Senkal M, Homann HH *et al*. Early postoperative enteral nutrition with arginine, omega-3 fatty acids and ribonucleic acid supplemented diet versus placebo in cancer patients: an immunologic evaluation of Impact®. *Crit Care Med* 1995; **23**: 652–9.

17. Senkal M, Mumme A, Eickhoff U *et al*. Early postoperative enteral immunonutrition: clinical outcome and cost-comparison analysis in surgical patients. *Crit Care Med* 1997; **25**: 1489–96.

18. McGeer AJ, Detsky AS, O'Rourke K. Parenteral nutrition in cancer patients undergoing chemotherapy: a meta-analysis. *Nutrition* 1990; **6**: 233–40.

19. Spapen HD, Duinslaeger L, Diltoer M *et al*. Gastric emptying in critically ill patients is accelerated by adding cisapride to a standard enteral feeding protocol: results of a prospective, randomized, controlled trial. *Crit Care Med* 1995; **23**: 481–5.

20. Moore FA, Feliciano DV, Andrassy RJ *et al*. Early enteral feeding, compared with parenteral, reduces postoperative septic complications. The results of a meta-analysis. *Ann Surg* 1992; **216**: 172–83.

21. Dobb G, Towler S. Diarrhoea during enteral feeding in the critically ill: a comparison of feeds with and without fibre. *Int Care Med* 1990; **16**: 252–5.

6

MECHANICAL VENTILATION

- Mechanical ventilation, especially intermittent positive pressure ventilation (IPPV), is the mainstay of modern intensive care practice and of fundamental importance to ICU therapy.

- Non-invasive positive pressure ventilation (NPPV) may be useful in patients with acute or chronic respiratory failure in whom invasive methods of ventilatory support are not thought to be desirable.[1]

- High-frequency ventilation (HFV)[2] has proved disappointing. Used in specialist centres to facilitate anaesthesia for airway and thoracic surgery but it seems to have a limited role in adult intensive therapy. Advantages include reduced airway pressures and therefore reduced cardiac effects, but outcome in respiratory failure has not been better than with conventional IPPV

Indications for ventilation

IPPV should only be used where there is a reasonable chance of survival. It should not be used as the last therapeutic act in a dying patient purely because it is available if it will only prolong the act of dying and the relatives' distress.

The prime indication for IPPV outside of the operating theatre is respiratory failure, but modern ICU practice recognizes the value of early ventilation as part of organ support in other critically ill patients especially in the presence of shock or cardiac failure.

Indications

Indications in the ICU include:

- Postoperative management, e.g. patients with morbid obesity, postoperative hypothermia, pre-existing lung disease, cardiac surgery and gross abdominal distension.

- Respiratory disease, e.g. pneumonia, lung contusion, asthma and other chronic obstructive respiratory diseases, and ARDS.

- Chest wall disease, e.g. patient with 'flail chest' following trauma.

- Neuromuscular disease, e.g. Guillain–Barre syndrome, myasthenia, etc.

- CNS impairment, e.g. drug overdose, trauma, status epilepticus, cerebral haemorrhage, tetanus.

- Cardiovascular disease, e.g. cardiac arrest, severe shock of any aetiology, pulmonary oedema.

- To provide organ support prior to organ donation in patients fulfilling appropriate criteria.

Protecting the airway against aspiration strictly requires tracheal intubation not IPPV but the clinical circumstances nearly always require IPPV as well as intubation.

The difficult decision is often not whether to ventilate a patient but more often *when* to ventilate a patient (apart from acute emergencies, e.g. cardiac arrest). This is difficult to be precise about and experience is often the deciding factor.

- Certainly gross hypoxia, e.g. pO_2 <8 kPa on 60% concentration of inspired oxygen, is a strong indication if there are no contraindications.

- Similarly, worsening hypercarbia and respiratory and/or metabolic acidosis are highly significant.

- Often trends of physical and physiological variables are more useful than absolute values.

- In accepting this one must not forget that hypercarbia usually develops relatively slowly whereas acute hypoxia can be lethal in minutes. It is better to intubate early rather than too late!

- General condition of the patient, e.g. presence of exhaustion, sweating, increasing restlessness or an inability to clear sputum, is important in indicating a need for ventilatory support.

Contraindications to IPPV

The decision to withhold IPPV in patients with chronic respiratory failure is difficult and requires the judgement of experienced practitioners. Ideally, the family and other professionals involved in caring for the patient should be involved in this decision. The patient's wishes should be paramount but unfortunately when the situation arises the patient is often unable to be rationally involved due to their illness.

In general, it may be appropriate to avoid IPPV (and possibly try NPPV) in patients with one or more of the following:

- Severe chronic respiratory disease with severe dyspnoea. Such patients are often receiving domiciliary oxygen.

- No identifiable reversible features.

- Poor quality of life, e.g. housebound, wheelchair-bound. Take care, as this is highly subjective!

Physiological effects

Cardiovascular effects

(The leading authority in this field is Pinsky and the reader is directed to his reviews in the Further Reading section for a full account.)

The two main effects of IPPV are:

- Lung volumes are increased – often significantly compared to spontaneous ventilation.

  - Large TVs causes a rise in pulmonary vascular resistance (PVR) which may lead to pulmonary hypertension and right ventricular compromise. This is due to the over inflated alveoli causing compression of the alveolar blood vessels. (Conversely shallow breathing, e.g. during weaning, can also increase PVR, partly by collapsing alveoli causing a fall in the diameter of extra alveolar pulmonary blood vessels, and partly by development of hypoxic pulmonary vasoconstriction.)

  - In addition, large TV leading to hyperinflation releases factors into the circulation depressing the blood pressure. Animal studies suggest these to be prostaglandins.

  - Hyperinflation can occasionally 'squeeze' the heart in the cardiac fossa causing falls in cardiac output (CO) analogous with cardiac tamponade. This is occasionally seen in severe asthma or emphysemas.

- Intrathoracic pressure (ITP) is increased at all points in the respiratory cycle – compared with the 'negative' pressures generated during spontaneous ventilation.

  - The heart operates as a 'pressure chamber within a pressure chamber' (as described by Pinsky) and it is therefore not surprising that changes in ITP affect cardiac function.

  - Thus changes in intrathoracic pressure are transmitted to the cardiac chambers during ventilation.

- Inspiration during IPPV increases ITP and therefore increases RAP relative to atmospheric pressure leading to a decreased gradient for venous return, reduced right ventricular (RV) filling and reduced RV stroke volume. In addition, the increased ITP decreases the gradient across the left ventricle that the left ventricle has to work against – this is one definition of afterload. In other words, decreased transmural pressure decreases left ventricular afterload. Both these effects tend to reduce intrathoracic blood volume.

- Conversely, with decreased ITP as occurs with spontaneous breathing during inspiration the opposite is achieved, i.e. decreased RAP, increased gradient for venous return, increased RV stroke volume, increased left ventricular (LV) transmural P and increased LV afterload. The combined effect is to increase intrathoracic blood volume.

- The decreased venous return and, therefore, decreased cardiac output with IPPV is the major haemodynamic effect of ventilation in most patients. As it is related to ITP it is worse if the ventilator is set to provide either a high TV (high-peak ITP) or a prolonged inspiratory time (high mean ITP). PEEP also exacerbates the fall in venous return.

- Venous return and cardiac output can be restored by either fluid infusion or sympathetic drugs both of which restore the gradient for venous return despite further increases in RAP.

Thus increased ITP not only reduces venous return (preload) but also reduces afterload on the heart due to effects on transmural pressure. Which effect predominates depends on several factors, e.g. presence of hypovolaemia and, most importantly, the state of the heart. Any beneficial effect on afterload in the normal heart is limited by the fall in venous return. In the failing heart cardiac output is relatively insensitive to changes in preload (flat part of the Starling curve) but exquisitely sensitive to small reductions in afterload. Thus, in heart failure there may be beneficial effects on cardiac output from increases in ITP with ventilation. In addition, it will be crucial in the failing heart to avoid large falls in ITP, as may occur during laboured spontaneous breathing, as this can dramatically increase both preload and afterload producing pulmonary oedema.

With high ITP, right ventricular afterload usually increases due to increasing PVR and development of pulmonary hypertension. Thus, high thoracic pressures can reduce LV filling due to RV distension pushing the septum to the left to reduce LV chamber size (known as interventricular independence). This effect of excessive high thoracic pressure can counteract the beneficial effects on LV afterload.

Thus the cardiovascular consequences of IPPV are complex and vary in differing disease states.

Respiratory effects

- IPPV causes a potential increase in V/Q mismatch due to preferential ventilation of the non-dependant, poorly perfused lung regions. PEEP in general will improve oxygenation by recruitment of poorly ventilated lung regions.[3]

- In the supine position FRC will be reduced due in part to upward displacement of the abdominal contents. This contribute to an increase in micro atelectasis.

- Decreased pulmonary perfusion if CO falls with IPPV causes an increase in alveolar dead space.

- Surfactant secretion is also reduced by prolonged IPPV.

Other effects

Humoral effects include an increase in ADH, renin–angiotensin and atrial natriuretic peptide lead to an overall retention of sodium and water. The oedema, particularly in the upper body, seen with prolonged IPPV is also promoted by inhibition of lymph and venous drainage from the upper body. The inhibition of venous drainage from the head may also result in a rise in ICP.

Beneficial effects

There is a considerable reduction in work of breathing and proportion of CO and VO_2 going to the lungs and diaphragm with a resultant increase in available CO and VO_2 elsewhere. There are some who think this is the only definite beneficial effect of IPPV. Other beneficial effects include:

- Improvement in alveolar expansion particularly where there is lobar collapse often secondary to progressive hypoventilation and exhaustion.

- Oxygenation usually does increase but not necessarily in severe pulmonary disorders, e.g. ARDS.

- Secretions are easily removed by suction or bronchoscopy.

- It is often only with IPPV support that adequate analgesia can be given to some patients, e.g. with multiple injuries.

Limitations of IPPV

- In general, IPPV does not reverse any intrinsic lung problem and is rarely curative.

- The ventilator should be viewed as adjunctive rather than primary support.

From the moment a patient is connected to the ventilator the goal should be to remove them from it as soon as it is safe to do so.

The results of ventilation are best when it is given as pure temporary support of the relatively healthy lung, e.g. overdose, hypothermia, postoperative patient. Results are not so good for patients with intrinsic lung disease especially if this is long-standing as there may not be any improvement possible in the long-term. The aim in such patients, therefore, is to support respiration while allowing time for other measures to be effective, e.g. antibiotics in infection, steroids in asthma. The results are worst when IPPV is instituted in conditions for which there is *no* specific therapy for the underlying problem, e.g. ARDS.

General care of the ventilated patient

- Airway: access via cuffed tracheal tube or tracheostomy. *Secure* the tube. Do not overinflate the tracheal cuff.

- Provide adequate humidification and clearance of secretions. The absence of humidification will encourage heat loss and dehydration of the upper respiratory tract. This can cause upper airway epithelial damage and difficulties with clearance of dry secretions. Conversely, excess heat and/or humidification can cause problems.

- Routine nursing care including care of the unconscious patient.

- Monitor appropriately. In view of the unpredictable and complex effects of IPPV on the circulation, be prepared to monitor the central vascular pressures and cardiac output. An arterial line is mandatory to facilitate blood gas sampling for all but the shortest periods of ventilation.

- N/G tube to relieve gastric distension and permit stress ulcer prophylaxis and nutrition.

- Ensure patient comfort as far as possible. For Sedation and analgesia, see Chapter 10.

- Ensure adequate nutrition and hydration.

Initial ventilator settings

- Set inspired oxygen concentration. 100% initially is sensible and will avoid further hypoxia while waiting for ABG analysis if there is doubt regarding the ease of oxygenation.

- Adjust inspired oxygen according to ABGs. Accept PaO_2 >10 for most patients.

- Set tidal volume at 7–10 ml/kg.

- Set rate at 10–14 breaths/min.

- Set PEEP if required. Most patients benefit from at least 5 cm PEEP if only to limit the required inspired oxygen concentration.

- Usual I:E ratio = 1:2.

- Usual inspiratory flow rate ~50–100 l/min.

- Continuous ventilation usually initially with pressure support if not deeply sedated.

- Set volume and pressure alarms.

- Set reasonable trigger sensitivity so as to be able to initiate spontaneous breaths if appropriate but so avoiding too sensitive a trigger which may trigger related to oscillations in the cardiac cycle.

All must be adjusted according to clinical response and frequent assessment.

Goals of ventilatory support

- Maintain oxygenation. The two main determinants of arterial oxygenation are the inspired oxygen concentration (obviously) and the mean airway pressure. This was first observed in neonates undergoing IPPV but was later observed in adult patients with ARDS.[4] Arguably, all other manipulations known to increase oxygenation, e.g. increased TV, PEEP, inverse ratio ventilation, exert their beneficial effect secondary to an increase in mean airway pressure. However, not all methods of increasing airway pressure may be of equal benefit to the patient, e.g. a minimum level of PEEP may be crucial.

- In patients with a profoundly low cardiac output, the low SVO_2 may also cause hypoxaemia.

- Recruit alveoli, i.e. open lung units and then keep them open. A low level of PEEP and a low TV avoids overdistension while preventing derecruitment of alveoli.

- Minimize complications of IPPV

Complications of IPPV

- Cardiac and fluid retention problems as mentioned above.

- Barotrauma and volutrauma (see below).

- Nosocomial pneumonia – for Antibiotics and infection control, see Chapter 9.

- Stress ulceration – see Chapter 18 on the patient with intra-abdominal problems.

- Complications of airway management (see below).

- Complications associated with ventilator malfunction or human error.

Barotrauma

Barotrauma strictly refers to any complication of ventilation related to thoracic pressures and could therefore include the cardiac effects. But most limit barotrauma to pneumothorax, pneumomediastinum, subcutaneous emphysema and the rare occurrence of systemic air embolus.

The mechanism is probably related to alveolar and bronchiolar distension leading to eventual airway disruption and interstitial gas formation. It is generally accepted that high levels of PEEP, endobronchial intubation and unilateral lung disease increase the incidence of barotrauma. Many now recommend that plateau airway pressures be maintained, where possible, <35 cmH$_2$O.[5] It has become accepted in recent years that 'low level barotrauma' can occur. Here, at low tidal volumes or in the absence of PEEP, repetitive opening and closure of alveoli cause damage from shearing forces.[6]

Volutrauma

It is now believed that in many acute lung disorders, especially ARDS, the disease process is non-homogenous, i.e. there are small, relatively normal areas of lung in conjunction with areas of diseased lung (known as the 'baby lung' concept). Put another way, in any one patient there will probably be areas of lung that cannot be recruited for gas exchange, areas which can be recruited with large TV and pressure, and areas of normal lung already recruited for gas exchange. If sufficiently high TV is used to recruit the diseased areas which can be recruited, then the normal areas will be over distended and damaged. Thus conventional IPPV may contribute to further parenchymal lung damage.

'Volutrauma' was coined to emphasize the role of excessive inflation volumes in secondary lung damage. Confusion arose because most early animal studies of barotrauma raised the airway pressure by increasing TV. A very elegant study examined pressure and volume truly independently for the first time (using a veterinary 'iron lung' to generate volume without increasing pressure and thoracoabdominal binding to increase thoracic pressures without altering TV). The authors clearly showed that histological lung damage only occurred in the high volume group.[7] Hyperinflation may also place the inspiratory muscles at a disadvantage by flattening the diaphragm.

Weaning from ventilation

- The most important indicator of readiness for weaning is resolution of the acute event which resulted in ventilation being instituted.

- During weaning the patient must have close supervision.

- The ability to wean is probably more related to the patient rather than to the weaning method used.

- Choice of weaning method is often based on personal preference and experience.

Various criteria have been proposed, the achievement of which predict readiness for, and likelihood of success of, weaning:

- vital capacity 10–15 ml/kg;

- tidal volume 4–5 ml/kg;

- spontaneous MV <12 l/min

- respiratory rate <45 breaths/min

- peak negative pressure, i.e. inspiratory force >20 cmH$_2$O;

- pO_2 >8 kPa on 40% oxygen;

- pH >7.3.

However, it is probably more important to satisfy several preconditions, i.e. the general condition of the patient is very important:

- stable cardiovascular system;

- no severe abdominal distension;

- no fluid overload;

- no major metabolic disturbances;

- adequate rest and nutrition;

- correction of pain and anaemia;

- cooperative patient.

An important study[8] examined various physiological predictors of the likelihood of successful weaning. Various indices related to oxgenation or the ability to generate pressures or volume were *not* useful. They found that the best predictor was the ratio of respiratory rate while temporarily discontinued from IPVV to TV (l/min). Normally this ratio is <30 (15/0.7 = 21.4). The study found that a ratio <80 predicted success while >100 predicted failure correctly in 95% of patients.

Weaning techniques

There are three main techniques generally available for weaning at present:

- T piece trials. The oldest method. The patient is allowed to breathe spontaneously for progressively longer periods as weaning progresses on a T piece system; returning to the ventilator in between.

- Synchronized intermittent mandatory ventilation (SIMV) – see Chapter 7. The patient can breathe in between machine breaths and the number of machine breaths is reduced as weaning progresses.

- Pressure support ventilation (PSV) – see Chapter 7. The amount of pressure support is slowly reduced until the patient is doing virtually all the work. A low level of PSV will compensate for the imposed work of breathing from the tracheal tube and inspiratory circuit.[9]

There have been two important studies comparing the different methods:

- one showed that PSV shortened weaning time compared with T piece or SIMV weaning;[10] and

- another showed that T piece weaning was superior over other techniques.[11] This is especially important for patients who have undergone a relatively short period of IPPV. An advantage of the T piece method is that it permits early recognition that the patient *can* breathe unassisted and thus avoid unnecessary periods of IPPV.

Despite the seemingly contradictory results, the overall message of these two studies is clear:

- spontaneous modes are probably best in patients with an intact respiratory drive; and

- whichever method is in use the patient needs to be observed closely, especially heart rate (HR), blood pressure (BP), PCWP and respiratory rate, and volume.

Weaning difficulties

There are many factors that may be involved in failure to wean:

- Increased work of breathing due to poor compliance, e.g. obesity, stiff lungs, bronchospasm.

- Unrecognized sepsis especially nosocomial pneumonia.

- Decreased ventilatory reserve, e.g. muscle wasting and fatigue, prolonged negative nitrogen balance, low serum magnesium, potassium and phosphate.

- Neurological causes of muscle weakness in ICU patients[12] may be a factor in the requirement for prolonged ventilatory support.

- Disuse atrophy of the respiratory muscles may occur rapidly.

- Increased ventilatory requirements, e.g. increased dead space, increased CO_2 loads due to burns, fever and excessive feeding with glucose and increased VO_2, e.g. due to shivering.

- Abnormal cardiac function (see below).

- Patent airway. Small diameter tracheal tubes increase work of breathing as does dried secretions in the tube lumen. Thus adequate humidification is essential during weaning. Tracheostomy may facilitate weaning by reducing dead space, facilitating secretion removal and improving patient tolerance.

- Ventilators. Increased work of breathing by the patient is required to open the valves on the inspiratory circuit with, e.g. SIMV. Also inability of the ventilator to provide peak inspiratory flow rates required on demand may be a problem. Older ventilators may also have an inadequate response time for cycling where the spontaneous rate is >30/min.

Correction of the above problems where possible may help the weaning process but failure to wean from IPPV is a difficult problem with no simple solution. Some patients who seem unable to wean may be helped by, and eventually weaned, using NPPV.[13]

Cardiac problems during weaning

The beneficial effects of IPPV on cardiac function in patients with cardiac failure have been alluded to. Much of the clinical evidence for this is indirect, i.e. adverse effects of discontinuing IPPV on cardiac function. The evidence is as follows:

- Patients with LVF and COPD may develop pulmonary oedema when IPPV is weaned with increases in PCWP from 8+/−5 to 25+/−13.[14]

- ECG recordings can reveal signs of ischaemia during weaning in many patients with coronary artery disease.[15]

- A careful study of patients with COPD but no identifiable heart disease demonstrated reductions in LV ejection fraction in all patients during spontaneous ventilation which was not apparent in those patients on PSV.[16]

- An important study showed development of a low gastric pHi to be highly sensitive and specific for the likelihood of failure to wean – presumably related to overall cardiac and oxygen transport deficiencies.[17]

The mechanisms proposed for these observations are:

- Increases in LV afterload with the decreases in ITP – especially if 'negative' intrathoracic pressures are generated during inspiration.

- Increases in intrathoracic blood volume as venous return increases with the decreases in ITP.

- Release of catecholamines during attempts at spontaneous breathing.

- Increases in the work of breathing, myocardial work and myocardial oxygen requirements.

- Increases in PVR with rapid, shallow breathing.

Thus diuretics, nitrate infusions and/or ACE inhibitors may all be temporarily required during weaning. It also seems logical in these patients to 'support' the heart with inotropic drugs during weaning. In many patients the cardiac status is the main limiting factor for successful weaning.

Iatrogenic ventilator dependency

A tracheal tube increases work of breathing. Generating pressure to 'trigger' the ventilator and allow a spontaneous breath requires 'work' – especially if the trigger is at the ventilator rather than the trachea.[18] It has been suggested that a too cautious approach to weaning may result in 'nosocomial respiratory failure',[19] i.e. tachypnoea during weaning may represent imposed work rather than patient work of breathing. In other words, tachypnoea is not always a sign of respiratory fatigue. If this is not recognized the patient may be placed back on SIMV or the pressure support increased rather than the correct response; which is to extubate the patient. The duration of ventilation thus would be needlessly prolonged with, of course, the likelihood of developing a nosocomial pneumonia leading to real ventilator dependency.

One needs to have a high index of suspicion for this situation and, perhaps, extubate when the patient is able to tolerate 10 cm of pressure support in a controlled but decisive manner as a trial of extubation.

Airway management

The choice is between oral tracheal tubes, nasal tracheal tubes and tracheostomy tubes. Each have their advantages, disadvantages and complications.

Oral tubes

Advantages

- Usually smooth atraumatic insertion.
- Easy suction of secretions.
- Familiarity.

Disadvantages

- Patient discomfort.
- Obstruction by bite.
- Problems with oral hygiene and mouth care.
- Laryngeal damage if cuff over inflated (reduced by low pressure cuffs).
- Occasionally difficult to secure, e.g. patients with beards.
- Dental trauma on insertion.
- Moulding at body temperature and movement within the oropharynx.

Nasal tubes

Advantages

- Better comfort, i.e. less sedation requirements.
- Easy fixation.
- Less oropharyngeal movement.

Disadvantages

- Sinusitus as occult source of sepsis.[20]
- False passages created during insertion.
- Bacteraemia on insertion.
- Nasal erosions.
- Epistaxis on insertion.
- Difficult for suction.
- Laryngeal damage – as for above.
- Longer than oral tubes – slightly increased work of breathing.

- Overall, most would agree that oral tracheal tubes are preferred to nasal tracheal tubes for most situations in the adult ICU.

Tracheostomy

Advantages

- May now be inserted percutaneously at the bedside.

- Best for patient comfort and tolerance.

- Less dead space.

- Best for suction.

- Easier communication, i.e. lip reading.

- No laryngeal problems.

- May be best for difficult weaning problem.

- Less accidental extubations compared with oral tubes.

- Not now thought to be associated with an increased incidence of nosocomial chest infections.

Disadvantages

- Some still require surgical insertion in theatre.

- Significant insertion complications, e.g. bleeding, false passage creation, damage to the posterior tracheal wall.

- Long-term problems with erosion into oesophagus or innominate artery late tracheal stenosis.

- Accidental removal may be a life-threatening emergency until track is well established (in ~48 h).

The indications for tracheostomy are controversial but include:

- Timing in relation to prolonged oral intubation (see below).

- Problems with sputum retention.

- Airway obstruction, e.g. due to trauma may be an indication for an emergency tracheostomy.

- An aid to weaning due to reduced dead space and work of breathing.

- Laryngeal incompetence, e.g. after CVA.

- A 'safe' inspired oxygen concentration so as to allow an adequate margin during the procedure.

Timing of tracheostomy   The question of timing after prolonged intubation is not always clear cut, e.g. tracheostomy need not be performed at 2 weeks if one is reasonably sure the patient will be extubated in the next few days. Conversely, tracheostomy should be performed earlier if one is certain that long-term ventilation will be required, e.g. for Guillain–Barre syndrome. The timing should be individualized in each case. There are no definite studies showing improved weaning with tracheostomy versus oral tubes but tracheostomy is associated with a reduced resistance to airflow and work of breathing. The shorter tube length may also be beneficial. One study did show a shorter duration of IPPV with early (<7 days) tracheostomy for trauma patients.[21]

Percutaneous tracheostomy   Insertion of a tracheostomy at the bedside using various commercially available kits has become standard on many ICUs. Costs are undoubtedly lower when including the costs of theatre time and time may be saved if one would otherwise have to wait perhaps several days for theatre time. Thus total duration of ventilation may be reduced with percutaneous tracheostomy if one looks at duration from the decision to insert a tracheostomy. Advances in safety and insertion technique have been recently reviewed (see Further reading). Studies are starting to appear showing a low incidence of late complications and improved cosmetic results compared with surgical tracheostomy.[22]

Removal   When the tracheostomy is no longer needed it may simply be removed. The stoma should then be covered with a dry, sterile dressing to provide a reasonable seal. Laryngeal competence should be tested prior to removal by deflating the cuff and giving the patient a drink of sterile water.

Minitracheostomy   May suffice in cooperative patients with problems with sputum retention. Routinely used in some centres to aid sputum clearance following thoracic surgery.[23]

Oxygen toxicity

Oxygen toxicity in critically ill patients is perhaps controversial but there is no doubt that in certain situations an excess of oxygen is toxic. (Before discussing oxygen toxicity one must not forget other hazards of high concentrations of oxygen, e.g. fire hazard.)

In general, clinical evidence for oxygen toxicity revolves around three situations:

- Oxygen convulsions (the Paul Bert effect).

Exposure to oxygen >2 atm may cause convulsions. The mechanisms are unclear.

- Retrolental fibroplasia (RLF).

The observation that hyperoxia is the major aetiological factor in the above condition has led to tight control of oxygen therapy in neonates. In rare cases a similar pathology can occur in adults.

- Pulmonary oxygen toxicity – of major relevance to ICU therapy.

There are considerable problems in investigating pulmonary oxygen toxicity, not least in distinguishing between the effects of hyperoxia and of the pulmonary pathology requiring ventilation. Many of the studies demonstrating oxygen toxicity were done on animals or human volunteers.

Certainly breathing 100% oxygen produces:

- slight respiratory depression;
- painful tracheitis;
- mild depression of both heart rate and cardiac output;
- constriction of blood vessels;
- with prolonged inhalation, depression of red blood cell formation;
- reduced secretion of surfactant;
- capillary endothelium permeability may also be increased leading to interstitial oedema.

In addition, inhalation of 100% oxygen leads to absorption atelectasis due to loss of nitrogen 'splinting' behind small airways blocked by secretions. This is a very real problem.

In the 1940s it became accepted that the threshold for safety was an exposure to an inspired concentration of 60% oxygen. However, convincing evidence is less forthcoming for two major areas of interest:

1. Causation of major parenchymal lung injury, i.e. the equivalent of ARDS.

2. Significant effects in ventilated patients with pulmonary pathology.

- In ARDS the systemic PaO_2 is usually normal despite the high inspired oxygen concentration. There is evidence that pulmonary toxicity may be related to high PaO_2 rather than inspired oxygen. During manned space flight, exposure to 100% oxygen at 0.3 atm produces no great problems.

- In cardiac surgery patients, short exposures (mean 24 h, range 15–48 h) to 100% oxygen was shown to have no significant clinical and radiological effects compared with a group of patients receiving a mean inspired concentration of 32% oxygen.[24]

- Another study, this time of irrecoverable head injury patients, found pulmonary changes, chiefly explainable by atelectasis, but no hyaline membrane formation as in ARDS in a group of patients ventilated with 100% oxygen for a mean of 2.2 days.[25]

Thus it is suggested that the mechanism of pulmonary damage in patients requiring high inspired concentrations of oxygen may be the associated ventilatory manoeuvres required for patients with significant pulmonary pathology, i.e. the high pressures, shearing forces and high lung volumes generated. In addition, some of the postulated harmful effects may be due to toxic oxygen free radicals. It has been suggested that a stepwise increase in FiO_2 (as is normally seen in the face of deteriorating gas exchange) results in the stimulation of protective enzymes, e.g. superoxide dismutase, that 'mop up' the free radicals, thus preventing many of the harmful effects.[26] Certainly there must be some protective mechanism at work or no patient ventilated with 100% oxygen should recover (and some eventually do).

In conclusion:

- Hyperoxia may produce harmful pulmonary effects, but it is very difficult to separate these effects from the effects of the pathology which necessitates the high FiO_2 in the first place or the associated mechanical ventilation.

- It is obviously sensible to limit the FiO_2 where possible (oxygen should be treated as any other drug with the correct dose being administered and unnecessary overdose avoided) to that producing the minimal acceptable pO_2.

- However, there is no excuse for allowing a patient to become hypoxic for fear of the risk of oxygen toxicity.

- The risks of barotrauma or hypoxia outweigh the risks of oxygen toxicity.

Further reading

Slutsky AS. American College of Chest Physicians' Consensus Conference on Mechanical Ventilation. *Chest* 1993: **104**: 1833–59.

Tobin MJ. Mechanical ventilation. *N Engl J Med* 1994: **330**: 1056–61.

Pinsky MR. Cardiovascular effects of ventilatory support and withdrawal. *Anaesth Analg* 1994: **79**: 567–76.

Pinsky MR. The hemodynamic consequences of mechanical ventilation: an evolving story. *Int Care Med* 1997: **23**: 493–503.

Friedman Y. Indications, timing, techniques and complications of tracheostomy in the critically ill patient. *Curr Opin Crit Care* 1996: **2**: 47–53.

Dreyfuss D, Saumon G. Ventilator induced lung injury: lessons from experimental studies. *Am J Respir Crit Care Med* 1998: **157**: 294–34.

References

1. Brochard L, Mancebo J, Wysocki M *et al*. Noninvasive ventilation for acute exacerbations of chronic obstructive pulmonary disease. *N Engl J Med* 1995: **333**: 817–22.

2. Froese AB, Bryan AC. High frequency ventilation. *Am Rev Resp Dis* 1987: **135**: 1363–74.

3. Ralph DD, Robertson HT, Weaver LJ. Distribution of ventilation and perfusion during positive end-expiratory pressure in the adult respiratory distress syndrome. *Am Rev Resp Dis* 1985: **131**: 54–60.

4. Marini JJ, Ravenscraft SA. Mean airway pressure: Physiologic determinants and clinical importance – Part 2: Clinical implications. *Crit Care Med* 1992: **20**: 1604–16.

5. Slutsky AS. American College of Chest Physicians' Consensus Conference on Mechanical Ventilation. *Chest* 1993: **104**: 1833–59.

6. Muncedere JG, Mullen JBM, Gan AS, Slutsky AS. Tidal ventilation at low airway pressures can augment lung injury. *Am J Resp Crit Care Med* 1994: **149**: 1327–34.

7. Dreyfuss D, Soler G, Basset G, Saumon G. High inflation pressure pulmonary oedema – Respiratory effects of high airway pressure, high tidal volume, and positive end-expiratory pressure. *Am Rev Resp Dis* 1988: **137**: 1159–64.

8. Yang K, Tobin MJ. A prospective study of indexes predicting outcome of trials of weaning from mechanical ventilation. *N Engl J Med* 1991:**324**: 1445–50.

9. Brochard L, Rua F, Lorino H *et al*. Inspiratory pressure support compensates for the additional work of breathing caused by the endotracheal tube. *Anesthesiology* 1991: **75**: 739–45.

10. Brochard L, Rauss A, Benito S. Comparison of three methods of withdrawal from ventilatory support during weaning from mechanical ventilation. *Am J Respir Crit Care Med* 1994: **150**: 896–903.

11. Esteban A, Frutos F, Tobin MJ *et al*. A comparison of four methods of weaning patients from mechanical ventilation. *N Engl J Med* 1995: **332**: 345–50.

12. Wijdicks EF. Neurologic complications in critically ill patients. *Anesth Analg* 1996: **83**: 411–19.

13. Udwadia ZF, Santis GK, Steven MH, Simmonds AK. Nasal ventilation to facilitate weaning in patients with chronic respiratory insufficiency. *Thorax* 1992: **47**: 715–18.

14. Lemaire F, Teboul JL, Cinotti L *et al*. Acute left ventricular dysfunction during unsuccessful weaning from mechanical ventilation. *Anesthesiology* 1988: **69**: 171–9.

15. Hurford WE, Favorito F. Association of myocardial ischemia with failure to wean from mechanical ventilation. *Crit Care Med* 1995: **23**: 1475–80

16. Richard Ch, Teboul JL, Archambaud F *et al*. Left ventricular function during weaning of patients with chronic obstructive pulmonary disease. *Int Care Med* 1994: **20**: 181–6.

17. Mohsenifar Z, Hay A, Hay J *et al*. Gastric intramural pH as a predictor of success or failure in weaning patients from mechanical ventilation. *Ann Intern Med* 1993: **119**: 794–8.

18. Banner MJ, Blanch PB, Kirby R. Imposed work of breathing and methods of triggering a demand-flow, continuous positive airway pressure system. *Crit Care Med* 1993: **21**: 183–90.

19. Civetta JM. Nosocomial respiratory failure or iatrogenic ventilator dependency. *Crit Care Med* 1993: **21**: 171–3.

20. Bach A, Boehrer H, Schmidt H, Geiss HK. Nosocomial sinusitus in ventilated patients: nasotracheal versus orotracheal intubation. *Anaesthesia* 1992: **47**: 335–9.

21. Lesnik I, Rappaport W, Fulginiti J, Witzke D. The role of early tracheostomy in blunt, multiple organ trauma. *Ann Surg* 1992: **58**: 346–9.

22. Fischler MP, Kuhn M, Cantieni R, Frutiger A. Late outcome of percutaneous dilatational tracheostomy in intensive care patients. *Int Care Med* 1995: **21**: 475–81.

23. Issa MM, Healy DM, Maghur HA, Luke DA. Prophylactic minitracheotomy in lung resections. A randomized controlled study. *J Thorac Cardiovasc Surg* 1991: **101**: 895–900.

24. Singer M, Wright F, Stanley L *et al*. Oxygen toxicity in man: a prospective study in patients after open heart surgery. *N Engl J Med* 1970: **283**: 1473–8.

25. Barber R, Lee J, Hamilton W. A prospective study in patients with irreversible brain damage. *N Engl J Med* 1970: **283**: 1478–84.

26. Crapo JD, Barry BE, Foscue HA. Structural and biochemical changes in rat lungs occurring during exposures to lethal and adaptive doses of oxygen. *Am Rev Resp Dis* 1980: **112**: 123–8.

7

MODES OF VENTILATION

P. Nightingale

This chapter will review:

- lung protective ventilator strategy;
- ventilatory techniques; and
- ventilator modes and adjuncts.

Although a large number of different modes of ventilation are available, it has been difficult to show that any one is superior to the rest. Using modes that allow the patient to breathe and those which are thought to minimize further damage, may improve outcome although more prospective studies are needed.[1]

Lung protective ventilator strategy

Mechanical ventilation is known to produce lung damage. Lung damage is thought to relate to:

- high end-inspiratory lung volume;
- repeated collapse and reopening of distal airways.

ARDS some lung units remain relatively normal (typically 30%) while others are collapsed, consolidated or fluid filled. The lung should be viewed as small and not merely as stiff. If volume-controlled ventilation is used with tidal volumes of 10–12 ml/kg, the relatively normal areas will be over distended leading to barotrauma.

Modern ventilatory management is to adopt a lung protective ventilatory strategy.[2] This is based on the concepts of keeping the lung open with positive end expiratory pressure (PEEP), but avoiding over distension by limiting tidal volume and end-inspiratory pressure. However, even if the respiratory rate is increased, this strategy may reduce effective alveolar minute volume and hypercapnia will develop.

Strategy includes:

- Maintain spontaneous ventilation wherever possible.
- Initial alveolar recruitment manoeuvres:
  - positional changes;
  - periodic sustained lung inflation (40 cmH$_2$O for 20 s).
- Adequate levels of PEEP to prevent alveolar collapse.
  - keep above lower inflection point on the static pressure–volume curve
  - avoiding 100% oxygen may prevent reabsorption atelectasis.
  - measure intrinsic PEEP.
- Avoid alveolar over distension
  - keep below upper inflection point on the static pressure–volume curve;
  - limit tidal volume (6–8 ml/kg); and
  - limit inspiratory pressure (end-inspiratory plateau <35 cmH$_2$O).
- Permissive hypercapnia:
  - allow PaCO$_2$ to rise if there are no contraindications, e.g. raised ICP.

This strategy can be followed using either pressure- or volume-controlled ventilation. Modern ventilators may now have modes that combine elements of both techniques.

Permissive hypercapnia

There are two circumstances where this is employed:

- In severe asthma low ventilatory rates (<6 breaths/min) may be needed to allow sufficient time for expiration to occur.
- In acute lung injury as part of a lung protective ventilator strategy.

In both these instances minute volume is often insufficient to maintain a normal PaCO$_2$. Although there are some potential cardiac and cerebral problems with permissive hypercapnia, at moderate levels (8–10 kPa) it appears well tolerated.[3] The acute respiratory acidosis does not require bicarbonate therapy.

Ventilatory techniques

Volume controlled ventilation (VCV)

VCV with external PEEP is the mode that has traditionally been used in the ICU.

Tidal volume (normally ~ 10 ml/kg) and heart rate (normally ~ 10 beats/min) are preset. Expiration is time cycled. Flow rate is usually preset (~ 60 l/min) and constant, although it may be possible to select a decelerating waveform. Tidal volume is guaranteed in the absence of leaks in the respiratory system, even if there are changes in airway resistance or total thoracic compliance. However, high airway pressures may be produced. The realization that high airway pressures were associated with barotrauma led to a degree of pressure regulation by setting an upper pressure alarm limit above which the inspiration was terminated.

PEEP

When airway pressure in the ventilator circuit has not returned to atmospheric at the onset of inspiration then, by definition, there is PEEP present. This may be set externally (usually in the range 5–15 cmH_2O), but intrinsic PEEP (PEEPi) may also be present. PEEPi occurs when there is expiratory flow obstruction, e.g. asthma, chronic obstructive pulmonary disease (COPD), or when expiratory time is too short, e.g. a rapid respiratory rate, prolonged inspiratory time. Newer ventilators usually have a means of checking the PEEPi level. It is important to note that the value on the pressure dial of a ventilator during expiration does not reflect the level of PEEPi.

When beneficial, PEEP increases functional residual capacity by alveolar recruitment. This reduces pulmonary venous admixture and increases PaO_2 at any given FiO_2. However, PEEP may produce unpredictable effects especially if lung compliance is dyshomogenous, e.g. consolidation in one lung. In volume-controlled ventilation (VCV), PEEP will increase peak airway pressure and may cause overdistension of lung units. Hence:

- Barotrauma is a risk
- Compression of vessels around distended alveoli may divert blood to underventilated regions, hence;
  - physiological dead space may be increased
  - shunt fraction may worsen
  - pulmonary vascular resistance may be increased

The preset tidal volume must then be reduced appropriately.

Pressure controlled ventilation (PCV)

With this technique, combinations of rate, inspiratory time, or I:E ratio, and pressure level can be set, according to the type of ventilator. Initially the pressure is set ~ 25 cmH_2O and I:E ratio $\sim 1:2$ or 1:1 in the patient with acute lung injury. Adjustments are made according to achieved tidal volume. Excessive airway pressures are avoided, but tidal volume will vary with changes in pulmonary mechanics. Small air leaks may be compensated for. Improvements in pulmonary mechanics lead to increases in tidal volume which may not be noticed since some ventilators do not have a high tidal volume alarm. In pressure-control ventilation, PEEP will lead to a fall in tidal volume, hence preset pressure or inspiratory time must be increased to compensate for this.

There are some theoretical advantages to PCV when compared with VCV. These include:

- regional overdistension/high regional PEEPi is avoided;

- peak airway pressure is lower for the same mean airway pressure;

- decelerating flow rate may be beneficial;

- alveolar ventilation may be improved.

Inverse ratio ventilation (IRV)

In this mode the usual set I:E ratio of 1:2 or 1:3 is adjusted by prolonging inspiration so that the ratio becomes 1:1, or greater. This theoretically allows for more even distribution of inspired gas to lung units with longer time constants. Because expiration is usually not complete before the next inspiration commences, air trapping occurs and intrinsic PEEP develops.

- Inverse ratio ventilation can be produced in VCV by an end-inspiratory pause or use of a slow or decelerating inspiratory flow rate, but there is a danger of an excessively high airway pressure developing.

- Inverse ratio ventilation is commonly employed with PCV by prolonging the inspiratory time.

- This may be safer than using VCV since high pressures cannot be developed.

Independent lung ventilation

By using a double-lumen tube it is possible to ventilate each lung separately using different modes and ventilator settings as appropriate. This may be useful in unilateral lung disease, e.g. the presence of one-sided aspiration, infection or broncho-pleural fistula. The ventilators do not have to be synchronized.

Modes of ventilation

Volume preset modes

Controlled mandatory ventilation (CMV)   In this mode, all breaths are mandatory machine breaths, and the set minute volume is delivered totally by the ventilator. The disadvantage of this technique is that if the patient tries to take a spontaneous breath or cough then not only is it very uncomfortable, but surges in peak inspiratory pressure are also produced.

Assist control (AC)   This term is used when the patient can trigger a mandatory machine breath.

Intermittent mandatory ventilation (IMV)   This mode was introduced to allow the patient to breathe spontaneously between mandatory machine breaths. It was thought that as mandatory breaths were reduced in frequency, the patient could add extra spontaneous breaths to maintain minute volume. However, the rate and timing of mandatory breaths were fixed, and once commenced, continued until the preset tidal volume had been delivered, with the potential for hyperinflation.

Synchronized intermittent mandatory ventilation (SIMV)   The technique of IMV was further refined to allow mandatory mechanical breaths to be initiated by, and synchronized with, patient effort. This added considerably to patient comfort with less need for sedation and paralysis. A problem remained, however, since patients with poorly compliant lungs tend to breathe rapidly. The increase in physiological dead space commonly seen in these patients meant that dead space ventilation tended to increase even though minute volume was maintained. Work of breathing could actually be increased if the ventilator was not able to respond fast enough to the patient's effort.

Mandatory minute volume ventilation (MMV)   If, during spontaneous breathing, the set minute volume was not going to be reached, then machine breaths were given. Unfortunately, when first introduced, the ventilator was not able to recognize the presence of rapid shallow breathing, and ventilation remained inefficient despite the set minute volume being reached.

Pressure preset modes

Pressure support ventilation (PSV)   When the patient takes a spontaneous breath, a variable flow inspiratory pressure is applied to the respiratory circuit by the ventilator. The level of pressure support should be set (usually ~20 cmH_2O initially) so as to give an appropriate tidal volume. Usually, airway pressure is maintained at the preset level until inspiratory flow starts to fall, at which point the expiratory phase commences. On some ventilators the level at which this occurs can be adjusted.

- This mode is now frequently used with SIMV as the mode of first choice for initiating mechanical ventilation.

- As with all triggered modes, it is vital that the response time of the ventilator is rapid or the patient's work of breathing can be increased dramatically.

- Newer ventilators have more rapid response times, often using flow-triggering, and the ability to control the rate of increase of airway pressure ('rise time'), thus reducing the patient's work of breathing.

Pressure controlled ventilation   There is a preset pressure that is maintained throughout inspiration and expiration is time-cycled. Flow rate is determined by algorithms in the ventilator and is initially high, to pressurize the respiratory circuit, and then decelerates.

- In clinical practice, for those patients with the most severe forms of respiratory failure, PCV is frequently used to produce intrinsic PEEP by prolonging the inspiratory time.

- Extrinsic PEEP is still required ($\sim$5–10 cm H_2O) to stabilize the remaining relatively normal lung units.

- Unless the patient is on a ventilator that allows spontaneous breaths, this method of ventilation is uncomfortable and this should be taken into account when prescribing sedation and muscle relaxants.

Airway pressure release ventilation (APRV)   This mode of assisted ventilation utilizes two levels of CPAP with the ventilator switching between them at a set time. The patient can breathe spontaneously at both CPAP levels, but the release of CPAP from a supra-ambient level to a lower level augments alveolar ventilation and hence CO_2 clearance.

- Typical initial values would be low pressure (5–10 cmH_2O), high pressure (20–25 cmH_2O) and I:E ratio of 1:1.

- Tidal volume is adjusted by raising the high pressure.

Biphasic positive airway pressure (BIPAP)   This mode is very similar to APRV. However, switching between high and low pressures can be synchronized with patient effort, and inspiration pressure supported. Essentially the mode can be considered as a variant of PCV, but allowing unimpeded spontaneous breathing at all times.[4] (BIPAP is a trademark under license to Drager and should not be confused with the Respironics BiPAP non-invasive pressure support ventilator.)

Mixed modes

With the development of more powerful computers, the electronic control of the newer generation of mechanical ventilators has become more sophisticated. It is now possible for ventilators to calculate the optimum ventilator settings and then allow breath-by-breath alterations in ventilatory support as necessary.

A number of new modes have recently been described, many of which are very similar in their underlying philosophy, which is to minimize airway pressure while ensuring an adequate tidal volume. This is now possible, in some cases, during both controlled and spontaneous breathing. These modes include:

- Adaptive support ventilation (ASV) and adaptive pressure ventilation (APV) (Hamilton Galileo ventilator).

- Pressure augment maximum (PAM) (Bear 1000 ventilator).

- Pressure regulated volume control (PRVC), volume support (VS) and Automode® (Siemens SV 300 series).

- SIMV^AutoFlow® (Dräger Evita series).

- Variable pressure support/variable pressure control (VPS/VPC) (Kontron Venturi ventilator).

- Volume assured pressure support (VAPS) (Inter7 ventilator).

The reader is advised to be familiar with each ventilator in use on their ICU by reading the manufacturer's literature.

Other modes

Proportional assist ventilation (PAV)   In this mode of ventilation neither flow, pressure, nor volume are set by the clinician! A gain control is adjusted to determine what proportion of the patient's inspiratory effort is supported by the ventilator. The term proportional pressure support (PPS) is used by Dräger in the Evita series.

High frequency techniques   These are arbitrarily subdivided into high frequency positive pressure ventilation, high frequency jet ventilation (HFJV) and high frequency oscillation. The rate varies from 60 to as high as 3000 ventilatory cycles/min. Since gas distribution may relate to airway resistance rather than compliance, it is possible to ventilate areas with both low and high compliance which are adjacent, e.g. a patient with ARDS and a broncho-pleural fistula.[5] Newer machines are capable of providing better humidification and are powerful enough to maintain lung volume in patients with ARDS.

External negative pressure ventilation   External negative pressure ventilation (historically provided by an 'iron lung') may be performed by applying a cuirass device to the chest wall. The Hayek oscillator maintains a negative baseline pressure to increase lung volume and oscillates around this.[6] There is a built in physiotherapy mode to aid removal of secretions.

Adjuncts

Tracheal gas insufflation (TGI)   Oxygen is delivered to just above the carina ($\sim$4 l/min) by catheter, either continuously or intermittently during expiration. The effect is to reduce anatomical dead space and increase CO_2 clearance.[7] The effect is to reduce anatomical dead space and increase CO_2 clearance and is more marked when there is permissive hypercapnia though there is obviously the possibility of excessive pressure developing in the lungs.

Further reading

Slutsky AS. Mechanical ventilation. *Chest* 1993; **104**: 1833–59.

Keogh BF. New modes of ventilatory support. *Curr Anaest Crit Care* 1998; **7**: 228–35.

Mehta S. Lung volume recruitment. *Curr Opin Crit Care* 1998; **4**: 6–15.

References

2. Stewart TE, Meade MO, Cook DJ *et al*. Evaluation of a ventilation strategy to prevent barotrauma in patients at high risk for acute respiratory distress syndrome. *N Engl J Med* 1998; **338**: 355–61.

3. Amato MBP, Barbas CSV, Medeiros DM *et al*. Effect of a protective-ventilation strategy on mortality in the acute respiratory distress syndrome. *N Engl J Med* 1998; **338**: 347–54.

4. Thorens JB, Jolliet P, Ritz M, Chevrolet JC. Effects of rapid permissive hypercapnia on hemodynamics, gas exchange, and oxygen transport and consumption during mechanical ventilation for ARDS. *Int Care Med* 1996; **22**: 182–91.

5. Hörmann Ch, Baum M, Putensen Ch *et al*. Biphasic Positive airway pressure (BIPAP) – a new mode of ventilatory support. *Eur J Anaesthesiol* 1994; **11**: 37–42.

6. Venegas JG, Fredburgh JJ. Understanding the pressure cost of ventilation: why does high-frequency ventilation work? *Crit Care Med* 1994; **22**: S49–57.

7. Petros AJ, Fernando SSD, Shenoy VS, Al-Saady NM. The Hayek oscillator. *Anaesthesia* 1995; **50**: 601–6.

8. Belghith M, Fierobe L, Brunet F *et al*. Is tracheal gas insufflation an alternative to extrapulmonary gas exchangers in severe ARDS? *Chest* 1995; **107**: 1416–19.

8

INOTROPES AND VASOPRESSORS

A cornerstone of ICU therapy is the improvement of one or more of:

- cardiac output;
- organ blood flow;
- organ perfusion pressure.

Improving the above *may* lead to a better outcome (see Chapter 1 for a fuller description). Failure to maintain the above is certainly a recipe for tissue hypoxia, multiple organ failure and death.

Some appreciation of the effect of stimulation of different vascular receptors will help understand the clinical effects of the commonly used drugs. Put very simply:

- α stimulation → vasoconstriction, some positive inotropic effect through cardiac α adrenoceptors.
- β1 stimulation → positive inotropy, positive chronotropy and arrhythmogenic.
- β2 stimulation → vasodilation, positive inotropy.
- dopaminergic receptor stimulation → ↑ renal blood flow, vasodilation.

Thus one would expect dobutamine (a drug stimulating β1, β2 and to a lesser extent cardiac α receptors) to increase cardiac output (CO) with some increase in heart rate and a minimal effect on blood pressure and noradrenaline (stimulating α receptors and to a lesser extent β1 receptors) to increase blood pressure (BP) mainly with some increase in CO and this is broadly what is found.

Two modern terms are:

- *inodilator* – a drug such as dopexamine or enoximone which has vasodilator effects and positive inotropic effects (either direct or by reflex owing to the reduced afterload on the heart); and

- *inoconstrictor* – a drug such as adrenaline with combined vasoconstrictor (often predominating) and positive inotropic effects.

Individual drugs

Dobutamine

Dobutamine is the inotropic drug of choice in most clinical situations – it is certainly the most studied in the ICU environment. Compared with dopamine it increases CO and stroke volume (SV) without significant increases in heart rate (HR) (and therefore smaller increases in myocardial oxygen demand) or arrhythmias. The competing effects of its two isomers on Alpha (L isomer) and Beta (D isomer) receptors usually result in only minor effects on MAP. As can be seen in Chapter 1, the increase in CO will result in global increases in DO2 to the tissues.

Dopamine

Dopamine is a naturally occurring catecholamine being the immediate precursor of noradrenaline. Its pharmacological action is generally dose-dependant but each patient's response may vary and, for example, harmful vasoconstriction may occur at quite low doses. However, in general:

- 2.5–5 μg/kg/min – renal vasodilation by stimulation of dopamine receptors.

- 5–10 μg/kg/min – β1 stimulation leading to increases in CO.

- >10 μg/kg/min – α1 induced vasoconstriction.

- The renal effects of dopamine are discussed in Chapter 16, but in general there is no convincing evidence for a renal protective effect in the critically ill patient.[1]

- The most common side effect, often at quite modest doses, is tachycardia and ventricular arrhythmias. Extravasation of the drug produces massive local tissue concentrations leading to vascoconstriction and necrosis.

- Compared with dobutamine, dopamine usually produces a lesser increase in CO and DO_2. Recent evidence of a harmful effect on pituitary function and an immunosuppressant effect[2] has limited its use in many centres.

Dopexamine

Dopexamine is a relatively new drug with predominantly β2-stimulating properties, i.e. is a potent inodilator causing only minor increases in myocardial oxygen consumption and negligible arrhythmias. In addition, dopexamine has significant dopaminergic stimulant activity.

- Recent concerns over 'renal dose dopamine' to preserve renal function have encouraged many centres to increasingly use dopexamine for this purpose with initial encouraging results.[3]

- Oxygen delivery can be increased with dopexamine with less cardiac adverse effects than can be achieved with dobutamine.[4]

- Splanchnic blood flow is increased with dopexamine and an increased pHi may be normalized.[5] The significance of this with regard to outcome is currently unclear.

- The use of dopexamine in high risk surgical patients as part of an overall approach towards oxygen transport (see Chapter 1) may improve mortality.[6]

Adrenaline (epinephrine)

Adrenaline is nature's own inotropic agent, active at all adrenoceptors. Adrenaline infusion results in variable inotropic and vasoconstrictive effects, with the vasopressor effects predominating at high doses. Most studies performed show increases in CI and DO_2 but no increase in VO_2 presumably because of a reduction in regional tissue blood flow from vasoconstriction. Harmful metabolic effects, e.g. hyperglycaemia and hypokalaemia, are more common with adrenaline than dobutamine and the chronotropic and arrhythmogenic effects can be dramatic. In addition, the use of adrenaline is associated with marked increases in myocardial oxygen demand because of its effect on increasing PCWP. Adrenaline is the agent of choice in Anaphylactic shock and CPR.

Noradrenaline (norepinephrine)

Noradrenaline is also a naturally occurring catecholamine with potent effects at α1 and β1 receptors. The associated vasconstriction predominates and limits its use to situations where increases in vascular tone are desired, e.g. septic shock. However, it is recognized that in septic shock noradrenaline may improve splanchnic perfusion by increasing a very low perfusion pressure[7] – providing the infusion is carefully titrated to avoid excessive vasoconstriction. Noradrenaline may also occasionally prove useful in cardiogenic shock to maintain coronary perfusion pressure.

Similar unpredictable effects on oxygen transport have been shown for noradrenaline as for adrenaline. Noradrenaline rarely causes tachycardia but excessive use results in tissue ischaemia and increased myocardial oxygen requirements.

Enoximone

Enoximone is a phosphodiesterase inhibitor that results in vasodilation, increases in CO and occasionally quite dramatic hypotension. It is not widely used but it may rarely be useful in shock with high SVR. The drop in MAP, even with careful titration of dose, limits its use. Enoximone differs from the above drugs in that it may be given as a loading dose (0.5 mg/kg slowly) followed by an infusion of 5–10 μg/kg/min. It exhibits positive lusitropic properties, i.e. it promotes diastolic relaxation of the heart – so-called inoconstrictor drugs may impair diastolic relaxation and worsen overall cardiac function.

Phenlyephrine

A pure α vasoconstrictor. Occasionally effective where noradrenaline has failed.

General points relating to use of inotropes and vasopressors

- Positive inotropic drugs such as dobutamine increase CO and organ blood flow.

- Vasopressors increase blood pressure. Occasionally noradrenaline increases CO but this cannot be relied upon.

- Positive inotropic drugs such as dobutamine do *not* increase BP directly. In fact, a slight fall in BP may occur due to vasodilation. Of course, this is usually more than offset by the increased organ blood flow.

- Positive inotropes such as dobutamine reduce CVP and PCWP by improving cardiac performance.

- Vasoconstrictors increase CVP and PCWP which may confuse interpretation of filling pressures and volume status.

- Titratability of all drugs discussed is made possible by their short half-life making them suitable for use by infusion.

- Digoxin is a weak inotropic drug with significant toxicity and its use in ICU should generally be reserved for situations involving tachyarrhythmias.

- Drugs with α effects should be given into a central vein. Peripheral extravasation of such drugs may cause tissue necrosis. Conversely, drugs without α effects may, in theory, be given peripherally although central access will probably have been achieved in any case for monitoring purposes.

- Data sheet infusion rates are only for general guidance only. All patients are different. The infusion rate of the chosen drug should be titrated to its clinical effect. The necessity for higher doses than is contained in the drug data sheet is commonplace

- This is best achieved by using a 'stock' concentration of drug in the infusion syringe and working in ml/h to a desired clinical effect rather than by working out the dosages in µg/kg/min (apart from intellectual interest).

- Very sick patients may suffer profound hypotension during even brief interruptions in the infusion, e.g. for changing the syringe. This can be minimized by *prompt* syringe changes (do not get caught out without a new syringe being ready) and usually prevented by either 'piggybacking' the syringe, i.e. starting the new syringe infusion a few moments before discontinuing the emptying syringe.

- Many believe that it is better to titrate specific drugs to specific effects, e.g. dobutamine to increase CO and noradrenaline to increase BP/SVR, rather than use one drug, e.g. adrenaline for both.[8] Although superficially attractive the use of adrenaline as a sole agent makes it difficult to achieve further increases in CO without excessive vasoconstriction – especially at high doses.

- The use of high doses of inotropes and vasoconstrictors without measuring their effects, e.g. CO and filling pressures, would be considered inappropriate by many practitioners.

- In the presence of hypovolaemia, positive inotropes can lead to serious falls in BP and marked tachycardia.[9] Therefore a fluid challenge may be appropriate prior to the use of inotropes in all but the most obviously overloaded patient. For similar reasons, inotropic drugs should not be prescribed unless hypoxia has been corrected. It has been said that oxygen is the best inotrope!

- Occasionally severe metabolic derangements may impair cardiac function. This may be correctable avoiding inotropic support. For example, severe hypophosphataemia may impair cardiac function – and may not be uncommon![10]

- Positive inotropes must be used cautiously in patients with ischaemic heart disease owing to the increased heart rate and myocardial oxygen demand associated with their use, which can exacerbate myocardial ischaemia and worsen outcome.[11] Realistic goals should be set consistent with adequate cardiac function and organ perfusion.

- An increase in CO may be more desirable than an increase in BP (i.e. an inodilator rather than an inoconstrictor). This is partly because the heart uses less oxygen increasing stroke volume than generating pressures, i.e. doing 'volume work' compared with 'pressure work'.[12] There is still controversy over whether the failing heart should be stimulated or unloaded, or both. Inodilators may do both.

- Nevertheless, organ perfusion pressure cannot be ignored. The heart 'likes' a low pressure (less 'work') – other organs do not, e.g. the kidney.

- Very low diastolic pressures may compromise coronary perfusion pressure, especially in the presence of tachycardia with its resultant reduced time for diastolic coronary perfusion. Thus, on occasion, noradrenaline may improve cardiac function by increasing coronary blood flow.

- Vasopressors such as noradrenaline may cause splanchnic vasoconstriction. If CO and filling pressures are maintained this is, hopefully, minimized. Certainly, appropriate use of noradrenaline, i.e. in patients who are well filled and have a good CO, improves renal function in the critically ill patient.[13] As added 'insurance' many practitioners infuse a small amount of a vasodilator such as dopexamine when moderate or high rates of noradrenaline infusions are used.

- Note: noradrenaline undoubtedly leads to renal shutdown in the presence of hypovolaemia.

- Prolonged (>72 h) exposure of the $\beta1$ adrenoceptors to stimulation results in a decrease in receptor numbers – so called 'downregulation'. Thus with time infusions of $\beta1$ stimulants such as dobutamine may seem to lose their effectiveness. Thus, increasing requirements with time to maintain a constant effect is not necessarily a sign of worsening condition. Conversely, weaning from quite high infusion rates may be relatively easy once the patient's condition improves. Downregulation does not seem to occur as readily at the α receptor.

- Prolonged infusions of vascoconstrictors such as noradrenaline induce a relative hypovolaemia by constricting the capillary sphincters. As the patient's condition improves the noradrenaline may often be weaned by 'filling up' the patient's vascular volume as the infusion is reduced.

- Positive inotropes increase urine output chiefly by improving CO[14] in addition to any direct effect on renal blood flow. This is probably the main way dopamine increases urine output.

- There often seems to be an irrational tendency once haemodynamic goals have been achieved to start weaning infusion rates immediately. Although it is clearly desirable to minimize the dose and duration of drug infusions, a period of haemodynamic stability and enhanced organ perfusion is probably more important. As the patient's underlying condition improves the infusions may cautiously be reduced but should be increased once more if there are signs of deterioration.

- The use of oral inotropic support to enable weaning of inotropic infusions has proved disappointing. Occasionally patients who are dependent on positive inotropic drugs can be safely weaned from such drugs using afterload reducing agents, e.g ACE inhibitors.

- SVR is calculated from direct measurements (see Chapter 1). It is irrational to titrate treatment to the SVR. In hyperdynamic states with a high CO there is no need for treatment if MAP is adequate – regardless of the SVR. SVR only needs to be treated if the MAP is low, i.e. SVR tells you how to treat the patient not when or how much.

Further reading

Feldman AM. Classification of positive inotropic agents. *J Am Coll Cardiol* 1993; **22**: 1223–7.

Barnard MJ, Linter SP. Acute circulatory support. *Br Med J* 1993; **307**: 35–41.

References

1. Vincent J. Renal effects of dopamine: can our dream ever come true? *Crit Care Med* 1994; **22**: 5–6.

2. Denton R, Slater R. Just how benign is renal dopamine? *Eur J Anaesthesiol* 1997; **14**: 347–9.

3. Downing HA, Ware RJ. Control of hyperkalaemia in acute renal failure with dopexamine – a new inotropic agent. *Clin Int Care* 1991; **2**: 336–8.

4. Boyd O, Lamb G, Mackay CJ *et al*. A comparison of the efficacy of dopexamine and dobutamine for increasing oxygen delivery in high risk surgical patients. *Anaesth Int Care* 1995; **23**: 478–84.

5. Smithies M, Yee TH, Jackson L *et al*. Protecting the gut and the liver in the critically ill: effects of dopexamine. *Crit Care Med* 1994; **22**: 789–95.

6. Boyd O, Grounds M, Bennett ED. A randomised clinical trial of the effect of deliberate perioperative increase of oxygen delivery on mortality in high risk surgical patients. *JAMA* 1993; **270**: 2699–707.

7. Meier-Hellmann A, Specht M, Hannemann L *et al*. Splanchnic blood flow is greater in septic shock treated with norepinephrine than in severe sepsis. *Int Care Med* 1996; **22**: 1354–9.

8. Levy B, Bollaert PE, Charpentier C *et al*. Comparison of norepinephrine and dobutamine to epinephrine for haemodynamics, lactate metabolism, and gastric tonometric variables in septic shock: a prospective randomised study. *Int Care Med* 1997; **23**: 282–7.

9. Shoemaker WC, Appel PL, Kram HB. Hemodynamic and oxygen transport effects of dobutamine in critically ill general surgical patients. *Crit Care Med* 1986; **14**: 1032–7.

10. Zazzo JF, Troche G, Ruel P, Maintenant J. High incidence of hypophosphataemia in surgical intensive care patients: efficacy of phosphorus therapy on myocardial function. *Int Care Med* 1995; **21**: 826–31.

11. Hayes MA, Timmins AC, Yau EHS *et al*. Elevation of systemic oxygen delivery in the treatment of critically ill patients. *N Engl J Med* 1994; **330**: 1717–22.

12. Noble MIM. Inappropriateness of 'inotropic' support with epinephrine. *Update Int Care Emerg Med* 1991; **14**: 81–9.

13. Desjars P, Pinaud M, Bugnon D, Tasseau F. Norepinephrine therapy has no deleterious renal effects in human septic shock. *Crit Care Med* 1990; **17**: 426–9.

14. Duke GJ, Briedis JH, Weaver RA. Renal support in critically ill patients: low dose dopamine or low dose dobutamine? *Crit Care Med* 1994; **22**: 1919–25.

9

ANTIBIOTICS AND INFECTION CONTROL

N. Randall

A point prevalence study[1] of European ICUs in 1994 (the EPIC study) found 45% of patients to have infections. Just under half of these infections were acquired in the ICU. The risks of infection come from both the underlying disease and therapeutic interventions:

- Increasing length of stay.

- Mechanical ventilation.

- Central venous catheterization.

- Urinary catheterization.

- Trauma.

- Emergency surgery.

- Organ failure.

It has been difficult to distinguish the contribution of nosocomial infection to morbidity and mortality. Selective decontamination of the digestive tract (SDD) reduces infections without improving outcome suggesting that ICU patients die *with* and not *of* infection. However, more carefully designed studies[2] have shown substantial increases in mortality (e.g. bacteraemia and pneumonia *double* mortality).

The EPIC study confirmed the increasing proportion of Gram-positive infections and the importance of the respiratory tract as a site of nosocomial infection in ICUs:

Organisms:

- Enterobacter 34.4%.

- *S. aureus* (60% MRSA) 30.1%.

- *Pseudomonas aeruginosa* 29%.

- *S. epidermidis* 19%.

- *Candida* 17%.

Site of infection:

- Pneumonia 47%.

- Lower respiratory tract 17.8%.

- Urinary tract 17.6%.

- Blood stream 12%.

The source of causative organisms seems fairly evenly divided between the patients' endogenous bacterial flora and exogenous infections related to various aspects of management of intensive care patients.

Deterioration in the condition of a patient should stimulate a search for a source of infection:

- Respiratory tract (see below) cultures.

- Blood cultures.

- Urine cultures.

- Review site and time of insertion of intravascular devices.

- Review wounds and drain sites.

- Intra-abdominal sepsis (including cholecystitis).

- Nasal sinusitis.

- Endocarditis.

- Infection of prosthetic devices.

- Central nervous system.

- Body temperature is unreliable – may be raised without infection or fail to rise (cool environment, haemofiltration).

- Leucocytosis is unreliable – suppressed by underlying disease or treatment.

Nosocomial respiratory infection

The ICU patient is prone to respiratory infection:

- Decreased sputum clearance:

- endotracheal intubation;

- inadequate humification;

- depressed cough reflex.

- Pharyngeal bacterial colonization (secretions leak past endotracheal tube cuff):

  - inability to swallow;

  - reflux of gastric secretions containing bacteria (antacid use, ileus, nasogastric tube);

  - sinusitis.

- Exogenous bacteria:

  - poor endotracheal suction technique;

  - contamination of ventilator tubing or humidifier.

- Pre-existing lung disease, including ARDS.

- Hypostatic infection

  - immobility;

  - abdominal distension.

Worsening oxygenation, increasing quantity and purulence of endotracheal secretions and new infiltrates on chest X-ray indicate infection. Tracheal aspirate culture correlates poorly with histological and microbiological pneumonia because of tracheobronchial colonization with bacteria not responsible for lower respiratory tract infection.

The most sensitive and specific diagnostic methods are from:

- bronchoscopic-protected specimen brushes;

- bronchoscopic bronchoalveolar lavage (6 × 20 ml saline) with specimens taken from a lung area identified on X-ray;

- each technique has a specificity and sensitivity >80%. However, interpretation of results is difficult in the presence of antibiotics.[3,4]

Central vein catheter related infections

- Central vein catheters (CVC) may become colonized by bacteria within a biofilm protecting them from antibiotics and natural host defences.

- Colonization increases with time, site of insertion (femoral > internal jugular > subclavian), and presence of a tracheostomy.

- The organisms are usually from skin (*S. epidermidis*, *S. aureus*).

- Bacteraemia rates as high as 14% have been reported.

- Subcutaneous tunnelled CVCs have much lower infection rates and PAFCs tend to be more frequently infected.[5]

- Diagnosis is by culture of the intracutaneous section of the CVC (cut catheter 1 cm distal to position at skin, rather than terminal 3–4 cm of catheter). Up to 15 colony-forming units (cfu) indicates colonization, and >15 cfu infection.

- Bacteraemia from a CVC is proved by culture of the same organism from peripheral blood cultures.

CVC infections can be reduced by:

- Skilled operator inserting CVC.

- Aseptic technique:

    - handwash, hat, mask, gown, gloves;

    - antiseptic skin preparation (chlorhexidine);

    - wide sterile field.

- Protocol for CVC care.

- Antiseptic or antibiotic impregnated catheters.

- Routine guidewire exchange of CVCs does not decrease rates of infection.

- Catheters should be replaced using a fresh puncture site when clinically indicated. As a compromise when access is difficult a suspect CVC may be exchanged over a guidewire and a new site used only if infection is proved.[6]

- Infusion solutions, three-way taps and blood-borne bacteria may also be sources for CVC infection.

Candida infection

Candida is an increasing problem:

- In the EPIC survey, 17% of patients had a deep *Candida* infection.

- Candidaemia has been reported to have an attributable mortality rate of 38%.[7]

- Culture techniques are improving identification of fungal infection. *Candida* antigen detection and polymerase chain reaction techniques should improve diagnosis. Fundoscopy may identify retinal abscesses.

Candida may spread to various organs (e.g. kidney, brain, eye) via the circulation and form microabscesses. Significant disease may therefore be occult. The risk factors are broad:

- artificial ventilation;
- CVCs;
- TPN;
- abdominal surgery;
- immunosuppresion;
- increasing severity of sickness.

The pattern of infection and clinical significance varies.

- Superficial mucosal infection of oropharynx or vagina responds to topical nystatin or fluconazole.

- Oesophageal infection – under-diagnosed but responds to oral and nasogastric fluconazole. Potential for progression to invasive infections.

- Urinary – common. Change urinary catheter and consider bladder irrigation with amphotericin.

The above three sites have little significance, except as markers of colonization. Systemic treatment is required for:

- Candidaemia. Commonly the result of CVC infection. Clinical state varies from no apparent effect to life-threatening sepsis. Any CVC should be changed using a new puncture site.

- Respiratory tract *Candida*. Diagnosis remains problematic because of *Candida* colonization of the respiratory tract without infection.[8] Mycelial forms in respiratory specimens and *Candida* from other sites, taken with the clinical situation, guide treatment decisions.

- Intra-abdominal *Candida*. A significant finding. Culture from abdominal drainage may indicate a continuing bowel leak.

- For *Candida albicans*, either amphotericin or fluconazole may be used. Amphotericin has to be used for *C. glabrata* and *C. krusei*. Amphotericin with flucytosine has to be used for *C.* meningitis and endocarditis. Change to amphotericin if there is no response to fluconazole.[9]

Methicillin resistant *Staphylococcus aureus* (MRSA)

MRSA is as pathogenic as methicillin-sensitive *S. aureus*, producing clinically significant infections (wound, lung, blood). However, MRSA is a much greater control of infection problem.[10]

Patients at risk of MRSA:

- increasing length of hospital and ICU admission;
- operation;
- antibiotic usage;
- artificial ventilation;
- CVC use.

Sources of MRSA:

- other patients (Note: transfers from nursing homes, wards or hospitals with known MRSA risk);
- staff (nasal carriage, hands, clothing);
- environment (bed and bed linen, adjacent furniture and equipment).

Transmission

- usually by contact, rarely airborne.
- strict control of infection measures are required to prevent outbreaks.[11]

Identification:

- evaluate risk;
- culture specimens from nose, throat, perineum, wounds, CVC punctures, blood, sputum.

Treatment:

- topical mupiricin for nasal colonization and small wounds;
- systemic treatment (vancomycin, teicoplanin) for more extensive/severe infection.

Vancomycin-resistant enterococci (VRE)

The problem enterococci (faecium and faecalis) have high level resistance to vancomycin (Van A and Van B types). Van B types are sensitive to teicoplanin.

Features in common with MRSA:

- similar patients at risk;
- similar environmental contamination; and
- similar transmission.

VRE differs because:

- affected patients are usually asymptomatic carriers;

- skin colonization a major problem, especially if the patient has diarrhoea;

- infections may affect gut, urine, CVCs, soft tissues and blood;

- some excess morbidity and mortality.

Clostridium difficile (CD)

The Gram-positive, spore forming bacillus is widely present in the environment and is part of the normal bowel flora.

- Clinical consequences variable

  - colonization;

  - diarrhoea/colitis;

  - pseudomembranous colitis.

- Detection of the A and B toxin more significant than culture of CD.

- Preceding antibiotic exposure usual but not invariable. Third-generation cephalosporins and clindamycin have highest risk.

- Treatment is with metronidazole or oral vancomycin.

CONTROL OF INFECTION[12,13]

Exogenous infections are amenable to some control by:
Unit design:

- 20 m² floor area per bed;

- 2.5 m 'corridor' space though unit;

- minimum one cubicle bed per six beds;

- minimum one hand-washing sink per two beds.

Unit operational policies:

- access of staff and visitors;

- patient admission;

- clean/dirty utility rooms;

- waste disposal, environmental cleaning.

Unit clinical policies, e.g.:

- nurse:patient ratios;

- staff clothing, hand washing, use of gloves and aprons;

- insertion of CVCs;

- use of ventilator circuits and humidifiers;

- endotracheal suction.

Infection control depends on staff compliance. Doctors are poorly compliant.[14]

Antibiotic guidelines

- Local policies should be developed and adhered to.

- Adequate specimens should be taken but treatment is usually started empirically.

- Antibiotics should be reviewed in view of clinical response and micro-biological results.

- Involvement of microbiologists is invaluable.

- Ideally, the narrowest spectrum antibiotic should be used.

- Treatment duration is debatable, but should be reviewed after five days.

- Dosages should be the maximum, tailored to body-weight and renal function.

Infection	Treatment	Comment
Community acquired pneumonia	Cefuroxime + erythromycin (or clarithromycin)	Reconsider if antibiotic treatment before admission. Benzylpenicillin if pneumococcal
Hospital-acquired (3–5 days after admission)	Cefuroxime or ciprofloxacin	Gram-negative bacteria more common. Add in metronidazole if aspiration may have occurred
ICU-acquired pneumonia	Ciprofloxacin, piperacillin-tazobactam or ceftazidime	Anti-*Pseudomonas aeruginosa* agent needed
Aspiration pneumonia	Cefuroxime + metronidzole	Upgrade cefuroxime if in-patient for >3 days

Abdominal sepsis	Cefuroxime + metronidazole	Initial treatment
	Piperacillin-tazobactam or ceftazidime, + metronidazole	Later treatment. Consider *Candida*. Surgical review
Pancreatitis	Cefuroxime or imipenem	Antibiotics only if necrotizing pancreatitis. Consider *Candida*
Biliary infection	Cefuroxime or ciprofloxacin	
Renal tract	Cefuroxime or gentamicin	
Meningitis (adult)	Ceftriaxone	Benzylpenicillin if meningococcal
Febrile neutropenic patients	Piperacillin-tazobactam or Imipenem	Consider CVC infections including *S. epidermidis* and *Candida*

- *Aminoglycosides:* efficacy dependent on high peak concentrations, higher peaks depressing bacterial growth for longer (post-antibiotic effect). Nephrotoxicity related to high trough levels. Once-daily dosing is a useful strategy in ICU patients whose volume of distribution and renal function may be fluctuating. Drug levels may then be checked prior to each dose.

- *Cephalosporins:* adjust dose if renal dysfunction. Third-generation drugs have significant bile excretion, disrupting gut flora. Ceftazidime and some newer drugs are effective against *Pseudomonas*.

- *Ciprofloxacin:* 400 mg i.v. twice daily for severe infections. Thrice daily regimens have been used. Well-absorbed enterally. Increases theophylline levels.

- *Imipenem:* formulated with cilastatin to inhibit renal metabolism. Convulsant metabolites may accumulate in renal failure. Meropenem does not have this problem. Appearance of *Stenotrophomonas maltophilia* a problem with both drugs. Imipenem concentrates in pancreatic tissue.

- *Fluconazole:* 5–10 mg/kg/day. Decrease dose if renal impairment, but double dose if haemofiltered. Do not use with cisapride (dysrhythmias).

- *Amphotericin:* 1 mg over 30 min as test dose then 0.5–0.7 mg/kg/day as 4-h infusion. Significant volume load. Wide range of problems so refer to data sheet or pharmacy before use. Monitor renal and hepatic function. Administered in a large volume. Consider colloidal or liposomal preparations, or fluconazole, if toxicity is a problem.

Acquired antibiotic resistance

Antibiotic usage is the overwhelming pressure for the development of antibiotic resistance. Control of antibiotic usage at individual patient, unit, hospital and, even, national levels will affect problems of resistance. However, resistant bacteria once they have appeared have proved much more persistent than had been hoped, and reappearance of multiple antibiotic resistance is likely when antibiotic pressure is reapplied.[15]

Further Reading

Widmer AF. Infection control and prevention strategies in the ICU. *Int Care Med* 1994; **20 (suppl. 4)**: S7–11.

Bonten MJ, Gaillard CA, Wouters EF *et al*. Problems in diagnosing nosocomial pneumonia in mechanically ventilated patients: a review. *Crit Care Med* 1994; **22**: 1683–91.

Reed CR, Sessler CN, Glauser FL, Phelan BA. Central venous catheter infections: concepts and controversies. *Int Care Med* 1995; **21**: 177–83.

Solomkin JS, Miyagawa CI. Principles of antibiotic therapy. *Surg Clin North Am* 1994; **74**: 497–517.

References

1. Vincent JL, Bihari DJ, Suter PM *et al*. The prevalence of nosocomial infection in intensive care units in Europe. *JAMA* 1995; **274**; 639–44.

2. Fagon JY, Chastre J, Viagnot A *et al*. Nosocomial pneumonia and mortality among patients in intensive care units. *JAMA* 1996; **275**: 866–9.

3. Bonten MJM, Gaillard CA, Wouters EFM *et al*. Problems in diagnosing nosoromial pneumonia in mechanically ventilated patients: a review. *Crit Care Med* 1994; **22**: 1683–91.

4. Wunderink RG. Mortality and diagnosis of ventilator-associated pneumonia. *Am J Respir Crit Care Med* 1998; **157**: 349–50.

5. Raad I, Darouiche R. Prevention of infections associated with intravascular devices. *Curr Opin Crit Care Med* 1996; **2**: 361–5.

6. Eyer S, Brummitt C, Crossley K, Siegel R, Cerra F. Catheter related sepsis: prospective randomized study of three methods of long term catheter mainte- nance. *Crit Care Med* 1990; **18**: 1073–9.

7. Wey SB, Mori M, Pfaller MA *et al*. Hospital acquired candidaemia. Attributable mortality and length of stay. *Arch Intern Med* 1998; **148**: 2642–5.

8. El-Ebiary M, Torres A, Fabregan N *et al*. Significance of the isolation of *Candida* species from respiratory samples in critically ill non-neutropenic patients. An immediate post-mortem histologic study. *Am J Respir Crit Care Med* 1997; **156**: 583–90.

9. British Society for Antimicrobial Chemotherapy Working Party. Management of deep Candida infection in surgical and intensive care unit patients. *Int Care Med* 1994; **20**: 522–8.

10. Romero-Vivas J, Rubio M, Fernandez C, Picazo JJ. Mortality associated with nosocomial bacteraemia due to methicillin resistant *Staphylococcus aureus*. *Clin Infect Dis* 1995; **21**: 1417–23.

11. Blumberg LH, Klugman KP. Control of methicillin-resistant *Staphylococcus aureus* bacteraemia in high risk areas. *Eur J Clin Microbiol Inf Dis* 1994; **13**: 82–5.

12. Intensive Care Society. *Standards for Intensive Care Units*. Intensive Care Society, 1997.

13. Ward V, Wilson J, Taylor L *et al*. *Preventing Hospital-acquired Infection: Clinical Guidelines 1997*. Public Health Laboratory Service, 1997.

14. Sproat LJ, Inglis TJJ. A multicentre survey of hand hygiene practice in intensive care units. *J Hosp Infect* 1994; **26**: 137–48.

15. Niederman MS. Is crop rotation of antibiotics the solution to a resistant problem in the ICU? *Am J Respir Crit Care Med* 1997; **156**: 1029–31.

10

SEDATION AND ANALGESIA

The two terms, sedation and analgesia, are often mistakenly regarded as interchangeable but should be considered separately:

- *sedation* – for hypnosis and anxiolysis; and

- *analgesia* – for pain relief and respiratory depression.

General points:

- It should be readily appreciated that being intubated and undergoing mechanical positive pressure ventilation must, at the very least, be unpleasant.

- Many of our patients will have undergone recent surgery and therefore will have painful wounds.

- Many of the procedures we perform such as vascular cannulation, wound dressing, physiotherapy, etc. also cause discomfort.

- The 'drive' to breathe against the ventilator can be reduced by appropriate selection of ventilator mode but constant 'fighting' the ventilator requires therapy to depress respiratory drive.

- Other advantages include less ventilator disconnections, decreased work of breathing and decreased myocardial oxygen demand.

- Appropriate sedation and analgesia will reduce the metabolic and hormonal responses to critical illness.

- Where dosages are described it must be appreciated that there is considerable variation between patients and development of tolerance sometimes necessitates much larger doses.

Much can be achieved by explanation and reassurance but most patients benefit from pharmacological sedation and analgesia. However, it is sometimes astonishing how well people tolerate a tracheal tube (particularly if the tube has been present for some time) with minimal sedation. Peoples' attitudes to sedation have also changed. In the early 1980s ventilated patients were deeply sedated and routinely paralysed with muscle relaxants. Now, with ventilator modes more readily interacting with the patient's own respiration, patients do not often require muscle relaxants. In addition, the hazards of excessive sedation are more appreciated, e.g. immune and cardiovascular depression, prolonged ventilator dependence, gastrointestinal (GI) stasis and cost.

Sedation

Patients in ICU rarely have a normal sleep cycle.[1] Attempts to maintain a normal cycle are important as lack of sleep or disruption of the normal circadian rhythm may be factors in the development of confusion or occasional psychosis seen in some ICU patients. Temazepam is an appropriate sedative to try and facilitate a 'normal' sleep cycle.

In patients undergoing IPPV there are several choices:

- Midazolam by bolus (1–2 mg) or, more commonly, by infusion (1–5 mg/h). In recent years there has been considerable concern that midazolam may significantly accumulate in the ICU patient, especially where liver function is impaired.[2] In addition, there is extensive protein binding and thus the action will be prolonged in most critically ill patients who have low serum albumin.

- Diazepam is too long acting.

- Propofol infusion (Start at 5–15 ml/h) results in much less 'hangover' and significantly shortens weaning time off the ventilator,[3] especially after short-term use. However, propofol is expensive and is not justifiable for every ventilated patient. Indicated where short-term ventilatory support is expected, e.g. up to 48 h, or may be substituted for longer acting sedatives after a prolonged period of IPPV to allow the longer acting drugs to be cleared from the system.

- Isoflurane for long-term ICU sedation is expensive, requires efficient scavenging and ventilators with vaporizers.

- Some practitioners use major tranquillizers such as haloperidol[4] to control agitation in ventilated patients.

- Opiates by infusion do contribute to sedation (apart from alfentanil which is almost purely analgesic and is a strong respiratory depressant) but their main use is for analgesia and to help the patient tolerate the ventilator.

Analgesia

- The use of regional blocks such as epidural or interpleural infusions may be extremely useful in the appropriate situation, e.g. chest injury, or after surgery. Epidurals are further discussed in Chapter 12. One should also, in most situations, use local analgesia infiltration prior to vascular cannulation even where the patient is 'sedated'.

- Morphine (1–5 mg/h) is commonly used and causes few cardiovascular problems when given by infusion. However, morphine has active metabolites and can accumulate especially in renal failure.[5]

- In renal failure the shorter acting (but more expensive) alfentanil should be used. Start with bolus of 5 mg and follow with infusion of 2 mg/h (maximum 5 mg/h).

- Tolerance to opiate infusions is common in ICU and occasionally their removal may be difficult with some patients suffering from 'withdrawal'. Relying on opiates on their own for sedation may not always be effective and coadministration of a sedative such as midazolam is often chosen.

Paralysis

- Paralysis is usually needed for intubation and suxamethonium (1–1.5 mg/kg) is the muscle relaxant of choice.

- Most ventilated patients do not need continued neuromuscular blockade to facilitate ventilation, but in certain situations paralysis is indicated.

- In general, the properties of atracurium (0.5–1 mg/kg/h) make it an ideal muscle relaxant for use by infusion and it is normally well tolerated haemodynamically. Requirements are reduced in hypothermic patients and increased in pyrexial and hyperdynamic septic patients.

- Routinely indicated only in severe asthma with high peak airway pressures, severe head injury to minimize increases in ICP with, e.g. coughing, and occasionally in patients with poor pulmonary compliance and critical oxygenation.

- Sedation should be assured to avoid the distressing situation of an awake paralysed patient.[6]

- Other problems include the inability to cough on suctioning (upper airway suction is inefficient at removing secretions in the absence of any cough) and a possible increase in DVT rate.

- Patients on infusions of muscle relaxants should regularly have their requirements checked with a peripheral nerve stimulator to avoid over dosage. Aim for one or two 'twitches' in response to a maximum stimulus of four twitches at 2 Hz.

Aims of sedation

It has been suggested that the goal of sedation should be a pain-free patient, who is clear, calm and cooperative during the day and who has sufficient restful sleep at night. This is difficult to achieve because:

- the 'ideal' drug does not exist;

- tolerance to agents is common;

- accumulation of drug is common;

- infusions are often increased, e.g. for procedures but often not turned down again afterwards ('ratchet effect');

- many nurses and doctors seem to prefer a 'flat', unresponsive patient.

In general, over sedation is more common than under sedation and less obviously, on casual examination, a problem. However, over sedation is not a substitute for reduced nursing staffing levels. Sedation should be for the benefit of the patient and not for the convenience of medical and nursing staff.

The disadvantages of over sedation include:

- more pressure area care required;

- decreased immune function;

- decreased cough;

- increased DVT;

- GI stasis (especially with opiates);

- prolonged weaning;

- increased risk of harm if disconnected from the ventilator;

- drug dependence and interactions;

- cost.

The use of a scoring system to guide sedative drug requirements rationalizes and formalizes the goals of sedation and probably avoids significant over dosage. It also can be useful to 'test' the degree of drug accumulation by occasionally switching off sedative infusions completely to assess conscious level. Of course, the infusion is recommenced when necessary; occasionally almost immediately (in which case there is no significant accumulation) but sometimes several hours later. This allows some clearance of excess drug and may reduce the amount of accumulated drug.

Numerous scoring systems have been developed – implying that there is no ideal scoring system.[7]

Further Reading

Park GR, Sladen RN (eds). *Sedation and Analgesia in the Critically Ill*. Blackwell Science, Oxford, 1995.

Shelly MP. The assessment of sedation. *Br J Int Care* 1992; **2**: 195–203.

Wheeler A. Sedation, analgesia and paralysis in the intensive care unit. *Chest* 1993; **104**: 566–77.

Pollard BJ, Bion JF (eds). Neuromuscular blocking agents in Intensive Care. *Int Care Med* 1993; **19 (suppl. 2)**.

References

1. Aurell J, Elmquist D. Sleep in the surgical intensive care unit: continuous polygraphic recording of nine patients receiving postoperative care. *BMJ* 1985; **290**: 1029–32.

2. Shelly MP, Mendel L, Park GR. Failure of critically ill patients to metabolize midazolam. *Anaesthesia* 1987; **42**: 619–26.

3. Roekarts PMHJ, Huygen FJPM, DeLange S. Infusion of propofol versus midazolam for sedation in the intensive care unit following coronary artery bypass surgery. *J Cardiothorac Vasc Anesth* 1993; **7**: 142–7.

4. Riker RR, Fraser GL, Cox PM. Continuous infusion of haloperidol controls agitation in critically ill patients. *Crit Care Med* 1994; **22**: 433–40.

5. Osborne RJ, Joel SP, Slevin MI. Morphine intoxication in renal failure: the role of morphine-6-glucuronide. *BMJ* 1986; **292**: 1548–9.

6. Loper KA, Butler S, Nessly M, Wild L. Paralysed with pain: the need for education. *Pain* 1989; **37**: 315–16.

7. Hansen-Flaschen J, Cowen J, Polomano RC. Beyond the Ramsay scale: need for a validated measure of sedating drug efficacy in the intensive care unit. *Crit Care Med* 1994; **22**: 732–3.

11

TRANSPORT OF CRITICALLY ILL PATIENTS

Transport of the critically ill patient is commonplace. There are three reasons for transport:

- Intrahospital transport, e.g. from the emergency room to ICU or from the ICU to radiology or theatre.

- Interhospital transport for specialist care, e.g. to paediatric or neurosurgical centres. (Note: this may be over long distances).

- Interhospital transfer due to lack of ICU beds

In all three situations the problems are similar and one should aim to:

- ensure airway and i.v. access;

- stabilize the patient before transfer, if possible;

- avoid last minute panic and rush. Planning should be such as to minimize delays and waiting in X-ray departments. Check the availability of equipment in the X-ray department before the transfer commences. Check that adequate porter services are available;

- continue current treatments, e.g. drug infusions, IPPV, etc.;

- ventilate with the same modes as in ICU. Modern, portable ventilators can supply PEEP and vary the I:E ratio;

- monitor for and treat new problems, e.g. arrhythmias;

- monitor to the same standard as in ICU;

- anticipate potential problems, e.g. extubation.

In addition, one must have the appropriate equipment including:

- portable ventilator;

- full oxygen cylinder (use ambulance O_2 – the cylinder is there for back up);

- equipment for reintubation;

- drugs – e.g. sedation, paralysis, cardiac resuscitation;

- AMBU bag or equivalent for ventilator/oxygen supply failure;

- suction (portable and ambulance);

- battery-powered syringe pumps if required.

Unfortunately problems are frequent[1] and may be a source of considerable morbidity. Transfer between hospitals by ambulance in particular can give rise to problems due to the cramped, claustrophobic conditions and the effects of motion on both the haemodynamic stability of the patient and the ability of the attendants to function.

It is well known that head injury patients will significantly deteriorate during transfer if inadequately resuscitated and the resultant secondary insults worsen outcome.[2,3]

Many of the patients will be intubated or ventilated. In general, members of anaesthetic or ICU staff are only required to be involved in the transfer of ventilated patients, patients with potential airway problems including comatose head injuries and patients under the care of the ICU.

Pitfalls and problems

- *Inadequate resuscitation:* Beware of occult injuries in multiple-trauma patients. If in doubt, intubate before transfer – the tube can always be removed at the other end if thought unnecessary.

- *Staff and equipment problems:* Inexperienced medical or nursing staff should not be used for transferring critically ill patients. Appropriate technical support should be available and should take a responsibility for the necessary equipment. It must be realised that some staff are not suitable for transfers if they suffer from motion sickness.
  Note: staff should be appropriately insured by their employers.

- *Logistics have to be addressed:* There is no excuse for battery-powered equipment becoming exhausted, oxygen cylinders emptying or drug syringes running out – even on long transfers.

- *Inadequate ventilatory support:* It has been shown that manual ventilation is unpredictable and unreliable compared with a portable mechanical ventilator.[4]

- *Inadvertent extubation:* Lifting of patients on and off trolleys is a cause of inadvertent extubation. It is probably safest to disconnect temporarily the ventilator for a few seconds during movement.

- *Post-transfer instability:* Critically ill patients are often unstable in the aftermath of a transfer.[5]

- *Hypothermia* – especially on long transfers.

- *Motion and its associated noise:* hampers communications, patient access and resuscitation attempts. If in doubt, stop the ambulance for resuscitation. In addition, acceleration and deceleration can lead to haemodynamic instabilty.[6]

- One needs to beware of *complacency* if 'only going down the corridor'.

- X-ray departments are notorious for problems developing with critically ill patients.

Further Reading

Pearl RG, Mihm FG, Rosenthal MH. Care of the adult patient during transport. *Int Anesthiol Clin* 1987; **25**: 43–75.

Guidelines Committee of the American College of Critical Care Medicine; Society of Critical Care Medicine and American Association of Critical-Care Nurses Transfer Guidelines Task Force. Guidelines for the transfer of critically ill patients. *Crit Care Med* 1993; **21**: 931–7.

References

1. Smith I, Fleming S, Cernaianu A. Mishaps during transport from the intensive care unit. *Crit Car Med* 1990; **18**: 278–81.

2. Andrews PJD, Piper IR, Dearden NM, Miller JD. Secondary insults during intrahospital transport of head injured patients. *Lancet* 1990; **335**: 327–30.

3. Gentleman D, Jennett B. Audit of transfer of unconscious head injured patients to a neurosurgical unit. *Lancet* 1990; **335**: 330–4.

4. Baxt WG, Moody P. The impact of a physician as part of the aeromedical pre-hospital team in patients with blunt trauma. *JAMA* 1987; **257**: 3246–50.

5. Waydhas C, Schneck G, Duswald KH. Deterioration of respiratory function after intrahospital transport of critically ill patients. *Int Care Med* 1995; **21**: 784–9.

6. Braman SS, Dunn SM, Amico CA, Millman RP. Complications of intrahospital transport in critically ill patients. *Ann Intern Med* 1987; **107**: 469–73.

12

THE SURGICAL PATIENT IN THE ICU

This chapter brings together many aspects of relevance to 'high risk' surgical patients admitted to the ICU – a 'pot pourri' of problems of the surgical patient.

Preoperative assessment

The aim of preoperative assessment is to minimize morbidity and mortality. Three questions should be asked when assessing surgical patients with the aim of minimizing operative risk.

- Is the patient's medical and physiological status optimum?

- If not, can the patient's status be improved (time permitting)? and should the operation still proceed? In other words do the risks of not operating outweigh the risks of operating? For example, medical status is almost irrelevant if the operation is clearly life-saving. Thus, no patient is 'not fit' for surgery – it just depends on the urgency of the situation.

Preoperative assessment should identify those patients who are at high risk of pre- or postoperative organ failures. Such patients may need additional monitoring and may warrant admission to ICU or a high dependency unit (HDU) postoperatively for organ function monitoring or support.

Patients are usually described as 'high risk' because of:

- respiratory disease predisposing to respiratory failure postoperatively;

- cardiac disease predisposing to myocardial ischaemia or cardiac failure postoperatively;

- less commonly, patients with renal insufficiency may develop renal failure postoperatively – vascular surgery patients are especially at risk; and

- one should not discount the effect of increasing age (see below).

Respiratory disease

The presence of significant respiratory pathology will lead to an increased morbidity and, for major surgery, mortality. Anaesthesia may not pose much of a problem but respiratory failure may result in the postoperative period. This in part will be due to the inevitable changes in respiratory mechanics associated with anaesthesia and the surgery performed.

- Respiratory excursion will be impeded by pain which may result in atelectasis.

- Pain may also inhibit coughing resulting in sputum retention.

- The site of operation is important, e.g. thoracic followed by abdominal sites being the worse – partly because these are the sites of incisions associated with most pain.

A review of preoperative respiratory function testing is beyond the scope of this text (readers are referred to standard anaesthetic texts) but certain risk factors are worth emphasizing:[1]

- presence of hypoxia;

- presence of hypercarbia;

- breathlessness at rest;

- smoking.[2]

The patient may benefit from being admitted preoperatively for:

- abstinence from smoking;

- bed rest;

- physiotherapy;

- bronchodilator therapy if bronchospasm present;

- antibiotics if infection present;

- nutritional assessment and supplementation if necessary;

- diuretics, if cor pulmonale present

Cardiovascular disease[3]

Presence of pre-existing cardiac disease is undoubtedly a predictor of increased perioperative risk. More specifically many studies have identified cardiac risk factors which include:

Previous MI	Left ventricular hypertrophy
Hypertension	Diabetes
Renal failure	Decompensated heart failure
Old age	Significant arrhythmias
Emergency operation	Severe valvular disease

Unstable or severe angina or electrocardiographic signs of ischaemia.

The overall message is that patients with severe heart disease and old and 'sick' patients are at risk of increased adverse cardiac outcome. Although anaesthesia can be problematic, most problems occur in the postoperative period emphasizing the importance of adequate monitoring and treatment of complications in the ICU in the postoperative ICU or HDU. Prevention of perioperative myocardial ischaemia is vital.

Prevention of myocardial ischaemia

The majority of perioperative ischaemic episodes occur in the postoperative period. However, perioperative cardiac instability (especially tachycardia) is a major risk factor.[4] Thus, anaesthetic techniques and problems are important. Choice of anaesthetic drugs is, however, relatively unimportant providing myocardial oxygen balance is maintained, e.g.:

- Factors increasing myocardial oxygen demand include:
  - tachycardia;
  - hypertension;
  - increases in contractility;
  - increases in wall tension (e.g. increased preload).
- Factors reducing myocardial oxygen supply include:
  - tachycardia;
  - hypotension (especially low diastolic pressure);
  - anaemia;
  - coronary artery spasm.
- Continuance of preoperative cardiac medications especially β-blockers is vital.
- Perioperative myocardial infarction (MI) (peak incidence on the second or third postoperative day) is commoner in patients with a recent MI but the incidence can be reduced by invasive monitoring and careful control of haemodynamic parameters.[5]

Oxygen transport in the high-risk surgical patient

It is well recognized that surgical patients may develop an intraoperative 'oxygen debt' as reflected by an inadequate VO_2, the magnitude and duration of which correlates with the development of organ failure and survival.[6] This oxygen debt is postulated to potentially arise from anaesthetic cardiac depression, direct anaesthetic reductions in tissue oxygen uptake, failure to maintain adequate fluid levels during surgery and perhaps hypothermia.

The best evidence for a beneficial therapeutic effect of maximizing oxygen transport is from studies where therapy was initiated very early in the presence of tissue hypoperfusion, i.e. preoperatively in high risk surgical patients.[7] Shoemaker's original prospective, randomized study demonstrating the virtues of optimizing oxygen transport was performed in surgical patients.[8]

The crucial message is that high risk surgical patients may have reduced cardiac reserves, especially in the elderly, suffer occult tissue hypoperfusion with a developing oxygen debt postoperatively, proceed to multiple organ failure if there is no intervention to reverse the tissue hypoperfusion and have a higher mortality than patients who do have sufficient reserves to reverse their oxygen debt and prevent serious tissue hypoxia.

A thought-provoking review points out that there are conflicting priorities in managing surgical patients at risk of myocardial ischaemia and those in whom the cardiac output and oxygen delivery need to be increased.[9] Both are at risk of an adverse outcome but the approach is different and identification of the group that patients belong to is important.

Fluid therapy

Generous fluid loading may be appropriate:

- Mythen and Webb[10] showed that fluid loading after induction of anaesthesia to a maximum stroke volume (SV) led to a reduction of the incidence of low pHi from 50 to 10%.

- Using Doppler ultrasonography to measure cardiac output (CO), Singer showed that intraoperative volume loading increased stroke volume and CO, resulted in a more rapid postoperative recovery and a reduced hospital stay in a study group of fractured neck of femur patients.[11]

- This approach must be tempered with caution in the elderly or patients with known heart failure due to the potential risk of fluid overload precipitating pulmonary oedema. Perioperative invasive monitoring may be indicated.

However, inadequate fluid therapy is more common, more dangerous (organ hypoperfusion leading to, e.g. renal failure) and less easily treated than the effects of excessive fluids which can, if necessary, be cleared with diuretic therapy

Importance of adequate analgesia

Adequate analgesia is important to minimize respiratory and other problems in the postoperative period. A recent study has demonstrated an improved survival for oesophagectomy patients managed by an acute pain service.[12]

Epidural analgesia has particular benefits:

- Improved respiratory function.

- Improved cardiac outcome and improved graft patency in vascular surgery patients.[13]

- Improved outcome and reduced costs in high risk general surgical patients.[14]

- Reduction in the hormonal stress response to surgery.

- Reduced DVT and blood loss for major surgery.

Combining an epidural with a GA may not achieve all the benefits of the epidural! There is some evidence that an epidural is not associated with decreased blood loss, rather GA is associated with increased blood loss, with or without an added epidural.[15]

Aspects of surgical nutrition

Current evidence would suggest that routine perioperative use of TPN is not indicated.[16] However, it may be beneficial in severely malnourished surgical patients. Enteral nutrition is always to be preferred where possible.

The morbidly obese patient[17]

Morbid obesity is a significant risk factor in the surgical patient. The main problems are:

- Increased incidence of hypertension and ischaemic heart disease.

- Mechanical respiratory problems, i.e. decreased compliance and functional residual capacity, especially when supine.

- Increased incidence of perioperative infection including wound and respiratory infections.

- Increased incidence of postoperative atelectasis.

- Increased incidence of abdominal wound dehiscense.

- Increased rate of DVT.

- Increased oesophageal reflux leading to increased risk of perioperative gastric aspiration.

Particular attention must be paid to assuring optimal respiratory function preoperatively and the patient should be warned that a period of postoperative respiratory support may be required. Important principles are:

- Extubate awake following full recovery of protective reflexes.

- Nurse upright – mechanical advantage leading to improved oxygenation.

- Need for supplemental oxygen in the postoperative period – potentially for up to 48 h.

- May be at risk for 'sleep apnoea' and this is exacerbated by the administration of systemic opiods.

- Epidural morphine provides better analgesia, faster recovery of gut function, earlier mobilization and improved pulmonary function compared with intramuscular morphine.[18]

The elderly patient

Surgical risk and ICU mortality is increased in the elderly patient[19] due to:

- Altered pharmacokinetics and pharmacodynamics.

- Altered physiology which can best be summarized as loss of homeostatic ability. There is a progressive loss of cardiorespiratory reserve (see monitoring strategies) and a loss of tissue elasticity. This leads to:

  - decreased myocardial and respiratory compliance;

  - decreased maximum SV, HR, VC;

  - decreased lean muscle mass;

  - increased work of breathing;

  - increased closing volume (may be greater than FRC).

  Many of these changes are minimal at rest, but increased during stress, including surgical stress. Thus with surgery or trauma, cardiorespiratory reserve may not be sufficient and failure occur:

In the kidney, nephron numbers fall leading, again, to loss of functional reserve and:

- problems with Na loading and depletion;

- problems with ability to concentrate or dilute urine;

- difficulty excreting an acid or alkali load.

- Increased incidence of concomitant disease. The above are fairly important but the increased incidence of significant pathology is very important in predicting increased surgical risk in the high risk patient.

Monitoring strategies in the elderly surgical patient

Invasive monitoring of elderly surgical patients has revealed a high incidence of 'hidden' abnormalities reflecting their reduced physiological reserve even in patients 'cleared' for surgery. Invasive monitoring during anaesthesia and in the postoperative period results in early recognition of problems, 'fine tuning' of cardiovascular parameters and an improved outcome.[20]

Postoperative hypothermia

Postoperative hypothermia has become recognized in recent years as a significant, and common, problem:

- Delayed awakening due to decreased clearance of anaesthetic agents.

- Most organ function is depressed by hypothermia.

- Haemodynamic instability during rewarming – increased fluids often needed as the patient vasodilates during rewarming. The hypotension thus produced can be confused with continued bleeding.

- VO_2 is increased by about 140% by shivering during rewarming.[21] If DO_2 not able to match this increase, the oxygen debt is prolonged.

- Wound infection may be increased by reducing skin blood flow.

- Hypothermia causes coagulopathy and a decrease in platelet count. Intra- and postoperative blood loss is increased with hypothermia; for example, the typical decrease in core temperature during hip replacement increases blood loss by ~500ml.[22]

- Adrenergic responses are increased postoperatively in hypothermic patients – responsible for increased cardiac morbidity. There is a 55% less relative risk of adverse cardiac events when normothermia is maintained.[23]

The degree of hypothermia in many of the studies cited was not that severe –35°C. Thus, development of hypothermia after prolonged surgery *is* significant and warrants management in the ICU. Forced warm air rewarming systems seem most effective for rewarming such patients. However, prevention is better than cure!

Further Reading

All major textbooks of anaesthesia will cover many of the topics included in this chapter. Also, there is a recent reference text specifically relating to the surgical ICU patient:

Hanson GC. *Critical Care of the Surgical Patient*. London: Chapman & Hall, 1997.

References

1. Nunn JF, Milledge JS, Chen D, Dore C. Respiratory criteria of fitness for surgery and anaesthesia. *Anaesthesia* 1988; **43**: 543–51.

2. Pearce AC, Jones RM. Smoking and anesthesia: preoperative abstinence and perioperative morbidity. *Anesthesiology* 1983; **61**: 576–84.

3. Report of the American College of Cardiology/American Heart Association Task Force on Practice Guidelines (Committee on Perioperative Cardiovascular Evaluation for Noncardiac Surgery). *Anesth Analg* 1996; **83**: 854–60.

4. Slogoff S, Keats A. Does perioperative myocardial ischaemia lead to postoperative myocardial infarction? *Anesthesiology* 1985; **62**: 107–14.

5. Rao TLK, Jacobs TH, El-Etr. Reinfarction following anesthesia in patients with myocardial infarction. *Anesthesiology* 1983; **59**: 499–505.

6. Shoemaker WC, Appel PL, Kram HB. Role of oxygen debt in the development of organ failure sepsis, and death in high-risk surgical patients. *Chest* 1992; **102**: 208–15.

7. Boyd O, Grounds RM, Bennett ED. A randomized clinical trial of the effect of deliberate perioperative increase of oxygen delivery on mortality in high-risk surgical patients. *JAMA* 1993; **270**: 2699–707.

8. Shoemaker WC, Appel PL, Kram HB *et al*. Prospective trial of supranormal values of survivors as therapeutic goals in high-risk surgical patients. *Chest* 1988; **94**: 1176–86.

9. Juste RN, Lawson AD, Soni N. Minimising cardiac anaesthetic risk: the tortoise or the hare? *Anaesthesia* 1996; **51**: 255–62.

10. Mythen MG, Webb AR. Perioperative plasma volume expansion reduces the incidence of gut mucosal hypoperfusion during cardiac surgery. *Arch Surg* 1995; **130**: 423–9.

11. Sinclair S, James S, Singer M. Intraoperative intravascular volume optimization and length of hospital stay after repair of proximal femoral fracture: randomised controlled trial. *BMJ* 1997; **315**: 909–12.

12. Tsui SL, Law S, Fok M *et al*. Postoperative analgesia reduces mortality and morbidity after oesophagectomy. *Am J Surg* 97; **173**: 472–8.

13. Tuman KJ, McCarthy RJ, March RJ *et al*. Effects of epidural anesthesia and analgesia on coagulation and outcome after major vascular surgery. *Anesth Analg* 1991; **73**: 696–704.

14. Yeager MP, Glass DD, Neff RK, Brinck-Johnsen T. Epidural anesthesia and analgesia in high-risk surgical patients. *Anesthesiology* 1987; **66**: 729–36.

15. Shir Y, Raja SN, Frank SM, Brendler CB. Intraoperative blood loss during radical retropubic prostatectomy: epidural versus general anesthesia. *Urology* 1995; **45**: 993–9.

16. Detsky AS, Baker JP, O'Rourke L. Perioperative parenteral nutrition: a meta analysis. *Ann Intern Med* 1987; **107**: 195–203.

17. Oberg B, Poulsen TD. Obesity: an anaesthetic challenge. *Acta Anaesthesiol Scand* 1996; **40**: 191–200.

18. Rawal N, Sjostrand U, Christofferson E *et al*. Comparison of intramuscular and epidural morphine for postoperative analgesia in the grossly obese. Influence on postoperative ambulation and pulmonary function. *Anesth Analg 1984*; **63**: 583–92.

29. Djaiani G, Ridley S. Outcome of intensive care in the elderly. *Anaesthesia* 1997; **52**: 1130–6.

20. Del Guercio LRN, Cohn JD. Monitoring operative risk in the elderly. *JAMA* 1980; **297**: 845–50.

21. Frank SM, Fleisher LA, Olson KF *et al*. Multivariate determinants of early postoperative oxygen consumption in elderly patients. Effects of shivering, body temperature, and gender. *Anesthesiology* 1995; **83**: 241–9.

22. Schmied H, Kurz A, Sessler DI *et al*. Mild hypothermia increases blood loss and transfusion requirements during total hip arthroplasty. *Lancet* 1996; **347**: 289–92.

23. Frank SM, Fleisher LA, Breslow MJ *et al*. Perioperative maintenance of normothermia reduces the incidence of morbid cardiac events: a randomised clinical trial. *JAMA* 1997; **227**: 1127–43.

13

THE PATIENT WITH MULTIPLE INJURIES

- Traumatic injury is the leading cause of death <40 years of age and the third leading cause overall.

- Traumatic injury is a common cause of admission to ICU – 16% of patients in one study.[1]

- Many patients are intoxicated.

- Injuries are often multisystem in nature.

- For head injuries, see Chapter 19.

- Chest injury is a common reason for the patient requiring prolonged IPPV and, therefore, chest injuries are discussed fully below.

Deaths from trauma follow a trimodal distribution

- Immediate deaths during in the first minutes at the scene are either due to massive haemorrhage or crush injuries, massive CNS trauma or (potentially avoidable) airway obstruction.

- Early deaths during the 'Golden hour' (see Chapter 2) are often due to the effects of haemorrhage or hypoxia and may be preventable

- Late deaths are chiefly due to sepsis and organ failure. Many may be preventable by prompt recognition of injuries and their physiological significance and definitive intervention.

DIFFERENCES BETWEEN HAEMORRHAGIC SHOCK AND TRAUMATIC SHOCK

Haemorrhage results in well-known physiologic changes. Traumatic shock includes these responses but they are modified by the tissue injury and its associated inflammatory response. This has several practical effects:

- Heart rate (HR) responds to haemorrhage by an initial tachycardia followed eventually by a progressive bradycardia.[2] This has been labelled as a 'paradoxical bradycardia' but there is nothing paradoxical about the heart slowing in the absence of adequate venous return in an attempt to maintain stroke volume. This *is* seen following, for example, ruptured ectopic pregnancy. With tissue injury there is no late slowing of the heart and tachycardia continues.

- Blood pressure is maintained by vasoconstriction until more than one-third of blood volume has been lost. With tissue injury, blood pressure is maintained to a greater degree by the surge in catecholamines and other nociceptive stimuli, but this is at the expense of tissue perfusion due to the excessive vasoconstriction.

- Animal studies show that, for an equivalent degree of blood loss, traumatic injury results in greater tissue hypoperfusion and a greater 'injury' than simple haemorrhage.

- The wound and fracture sites are metabolically active with a resultant requirement for increased oxygen consumption and glucose oxidation – the concept of 'the wound as an organ'.[3] In addition to the local reasons for increased metabolic demands, there are systemic inflammatory and catabolic causes of increased metabolic demand requiring an increased cardiac output compared with normal. This may have implications for therapy.

ASSESSMENT OF THE TRAUMA PATIENT

- A system for evaluation of trauma victims results in faster, more effective resuscitation, fewer life-threatening injuries missed and a greater appreciation of priorities.

- The Advanced Trauma Life Support system, as promoted by the American College of Surgeons since 1979, is one such system that has gained widespread acceptance.

- Assessment, diagnosis and initial treatment should be carried out simultaneously.

- This is facilitated by a team approach with a 'team leader'.

- The patient needs to be completely undressed and examined thoroughly as blunt, high-velocity injury can result in injury to virtually any part of the body.

- The first priorities are to detect and treat immediately life-threatening conditions while second priorities are to detect other injuries (none should be missed).

- Radiological investigations should not take priority over resuscitation.

- Relevant senior specialists should be involved at an early stage.

- Someone experienced should evaluate the abdomen. Peritoneal lavage may be performed where doubt exists regarding the presence of an intra-abdominal injury. Abdominal ultrasound or CT scanning have their advocates.

- Do not forget to administer appropriate antibiotics and tetanus toxoid.

- All dislocations and fractures should be splinted and reduced if possible. This eases nursing, reduces pain and bleeding, and may reduce the incidence of ARDS (see below).

RESUSCITATION

The ABC system is widely followed:

- A = airway including cervical spine protection;

- B = breathing;

- C = circulation;

- D = disability/neurological assessment including GCS;

- E = exposure – undress completely.

The less well-known system of VIP (ventilation, infusion and perfusion) is perhaps more appropriate for trauma patients[4] as it emphasizes the inter-relationship between ventilation and perfusion in overall oxygen transport and because it reminds us that the cornerstone of resuscitation of victims of traumatic injury is fluid infusion.

Airway and cervical spine protection[5]

- The airway *must* be clear or permanent neurological damage or death may occur in minutes.

- The cervical spine should be assumed to be at risk and protected from further damage until proven by radiological screening to be intact. A hard cervical collar is mandatory.

- Unless immediate intubation is required the cervical spine should be assessed by adequate radiological views of all seven cervical vertebrae. One should look for:

  - normal soft tissue shadows;

  - normal vertebral alignment; and

  - normal cervical lordosis.

- If intubation is required, the technique of choice is preoxygenation followed by oral intubation with manual in-line stabilization of the cervical spine by an assistant. Cricoid pressure to reduce the risk of aspiration of stomach contents should be performed.

- It is difficult to find good evidence that this technique, properly performed, has resulted in *additional* neurological impairment in any trauma patient with cervical spine injury. Neurological signs should be documented before intubation, if possible.

- Alternative approaches are impractical or associated with increased complications, e.g.:

Fibreoptic awake intubation	nasal intubation;
unfamiliar technique practitioners	for most increased failure rate; epistaxis;
uncooperative or obtunded patient	bacteraemia; potentially greater C spine movement.

- If the patient cannot be intubated then a surgical airway should be created, i.e. cricothrotomy.

Breathing/ventilation

- High flow O_2 should be administered to all patients.

- Clinically obvious pneumothoraces should be drained.

- There should be an extremely low threshold for immediate tracheal intubation on clinical grounds – even before the result of arterial blood gases.

- Indications for immediate intubation and ventilation include gross respiratory distress, obvious hypoventilation and severe shock.

- Delayed ventilation by promoting tissue hypoxia results in an increased incidence of organ failures.

Circulation

- External haemorrhage must be controlled.

- Large bore catheters (X2) are inserted and volume infused.

- All multiple-injured patients should have large volumes of warmed i.v. fluids, administered quickly.

- One is far more likely to run into problems of inadequate infusion than problems of excess infusion.

- As soon as possible, blood should be sent for blood gas analysis and cross-matching.

Infusion

- The choice of fluid is controversial. For the 'colloid/crystalloid' debate, see Chapter 4. However, what *can* be stated with certainty is that multiple-trauma patients will almost certainly require the transfusion of blood.

- Crystalloid solution (2 litres) or colloid (1 litre) should be administered as rapidly as possible in any multiple-injured patient followed by further fluids including blood as indicated.

- Be prepared to give type-specific but uncross-matched blood or O-negative blood *in extremis*.

- Many junior doctors do not appreciate the magnitude of concealed blood loss from closed orthopaedic injuries, e.g. 2 litres from a femoral shaft fracture and potential exsanguination from a bad pelvic fracture.

- In all but the most desperate situations, the skin should be appropriately prepared prior to venous cannulation as the leading cause of late death in trauma patients is sepsis.

- In cases of massive blood loss and transfusion, maintenance of coagulation must be addressed and infusions of FFP and platelets given as indicated by results of coagulation screens.

Permissive hypovolaemia

- An important study in 1994 of penetrating trauma showed an improved survival in those patients with 'delayed' fluid resuscitation, i.e. minimal i.v. fluids given prior to definitive operative intervention.[6] This has been called 'permissive hypovolaemia'.

- The rationale, suggested by previous animal studies, is that full resuscitation results in:

  - a higher BP disrupting clot formation;

  - haemodilution and decreased viscosity disrupt clot formation;

  - dilutional coagulopathy.

- The recommendation has, therefore, been made to limit fluids to maintain a MAP ≤ 50 until bleeding has been surgically controlled, *then* proceed to full resuscitation.

- The problems limiting widespread acceptance of this concept are:

  - the need for *prompt* definitive intervention to minimize the oxygen debt;

  - delays in surgery, e.g. in rural area may be better with 'normal' resuscitation;

  - this approach is inappropriate for patients who also have head injury.

- The biggest problem is that this study was performed in *penetrating* injuries. Patients with blunt trauma (the majority) are not so likely to have definitive surgical interventions.

Differences between blunt and penetrating trauma

Penetrating:

- Common in the USA.

- Often sole injury.

- Diagnosis often simple.

- Surgery often definitive treatment.

Blunt:

- More common in Europe.

- Not usually in isolation.

- Diagnosis often complex.

- Surgery rarely definitive.

- Therefore, this approach is not recommended in patients suffering blunt trauma.

- Further controlled trials are awaited but it would be unfortunate if improvements in trauma management related to an understanding of the importance of rapid resuscitation (the 'Golden hour' concept) with volume infusion as a cornerstone of that resuscitation were lost because fluid restriction was seen as appropriate in any but a few specific (and uncommon) circumstances.

Perfusion

- The overall goal of all resuscitation procedures is to improve oxygenation and perfusion of body tissues.

- Oxygen therapy and maintenance of blood volume and oxygen-carrying capacity is usually sufficient to restore homeostasis in the majority of trauma victims.

- It is worth remembering that even in the young patient cardiac function can be severely compromised in haemorrhagic shock so that an element of cardiogenic shock contributes to the shocked state. In such cases the response to resuscitation may be compromised and invasive monitoring and/or inotropes required as detailed below.

- As early as the 1950s the contribution of the heart to progressive, irreversible shock was recognized and it was also demonstrated that the homeostatic mechanisms and vasoconstriction were not sufficient to maintain coronary perfusion in severe haemorrhage.

- Therefore, cardiac dysfunction needs to be detected and corrected as early after injury as possible.

Goals of resuscitation

- In most uncomplicated cases where resuscitation has been rapid the goals of resuscitation are:

Increase:

- BP

- Urine output

- Capillary perfusion

- Conscious level

Decrease:

- HR

- Temperature

- Increases in urine output and conscious level are assumed to reflect increased organ perfusion overall.

- Invasive haemodynamic monitoring with a pulmonary artery catheter is not required in most patients.

- However, *all* patients who do not respond promptly to oxygenation and volume resuscitation with or without surgery should be invasively monitored to guide optimal fluid therapy and detect cardiac dysfunction.

- The threshold for invasive monitoring should be lower in the elderly patient and those with existing disease states.

The rationale for a low threshold for invasive monitoring is as follows:

Problems of inadequate cardiac output and occult shock

One study in the elderly[7] emphasized the importance of early detection of cardiac dysfunction by invasive monitoring using a PAFC. Elderly trauma patients who had low cardiac output who were on average monitored 5.5 h after injury had an overall survival of only 7% – the rest dying of cardiogenic shock and multiple organ failure. Thirty similar elderly patients were then studied. These patients were monitored much earlier – in a mean time of 2.2 h. Low cardiac outputs were detected, inotropic support provided and the overall survival in this second similar group was 53%. The message is clear:

- Elderly trauma patients may have dangerously low cardiac output unrecognized by non-invasive monitoring. If this is left untreated cardiogenic shock and organ failure may supervene. It is interesting to compare the results of this study with the largely empirical idea of the 'Golden hour'.

- Further studies on younger patients have shown similar results with similar conclusions.[8]

Problems with BP and HR as indices of resuscitation

Fluid therapy regimens have been promoted relying on changes in HR and blood pressure (BP) to guide fluid requirements. This is not an adequate approach for all patients. Heart rate and MAP are affected by the degree of tissue trauma as well as the degree of hypovolaemia.[2] In addition, studies show[9] poor correlation between MAP and CI:

- HR and changes in HR poorly correlate with CI.

- MAP and CI only correlated well at initial measurement and preterminally.

- By the time hypovolaemia and low CI are of sufficient magnitude to produce hypotension their correlation is greatly improved, but by this time the deteriorating circulating condition is well advanced. Therefore, reliance on hypotension as an early warning sign of shock or reliance on a normal BP as a measure of adequate fluid resuscitation or tissue perfusion may be unwarranted.

Indices of adequate resuscitation

The goals of resuscitation in complicated or prolonged resuscitations include:

- Optimal CI with optimal PCWP.

- Normal lactate and base deficit (BD). The time needed to normalize serum lactate levels is an important prognostic factor for survival in the severely injured patient. BD correlates well with degree of injury, magnitude of blood loss and outcome.[10] In a laboratory model, the BD was superior to any other measurable parameter in identifying degree of haemorrhage.[11]

- Supranormal oxygen transport goals. While there is doubt about the general applicability of attempting to achieve 'supranormal' CI, DO_2 and VO_2 in all ICU patients, there is still convincing evidence for their usefulness in traumatic injury. For example:

  - reaching supranormal circulatory values, especially in 24 h of injury, may improve survival and reduce the frequency of shock-related organ failure in the severely traumatized patient;[12] and

  - increased CI, DO_2, and VO_2 seen in survivors of severe trauma are primary compensations that have survival value; augmentation of these compensations compared with conventional therapy decreases mortality.[13]

  Possible reasons for the value of this approach include the concept of 'the wound as an organ'.

  Only one major study has failed to find evidence of benefit from achieving supranormal goals.[14]

- pHi. This may be an important marker to assess the adequacy of resuscitation. pHi monitoring may provide early warning for systemic complications in the postresuscitation period.[15]

Operative intervention

- Many trauma patients will need surgery.

- In general, all the required surgical procedures should be performed acutely, i.e. during one anaesthetic providing the patient has been appropriately resuscitated and is haemodynamically stable.

- The rationale is that once the patient is resuscitated, they will be in the best condition that s/he will be in for some time, i.e. before the development of sepsis, tissue oedema, malnutrition and metabolic complications.

- Delayed fixation of long bone fractures may increase the incidence of ARDS.[16] The mechanisms are uncertain but will probably include ongoing bleeding, increased pain, and physiological stress response and possible fat embolus.

- Conversely if the patient undergoing surgery *is* unstable with developing hypothermia, coagulopathy and acidosis, prolonged surgery has a high mortality rate. Many surgeons now accept that the best way to manage these patients is to 'bail out', e.g. pack the abdomen to stop bleeding, bring out bowel the ends on to the abdominal wall, etc., and to take the patient to ICU for stabilization and further resuscitation. Further surgical intervention is deferred to a later date. This has been described as 'damage control surgery'.[17]

Chest injuries

Immediate management:

- Ensure a patent airway.

- Administer oxygen.

- Exclude:

  - pneumothorax;

  - haemothorax;

  - cardiac tamponade.

- Emergency management of tension pneumothorax with either severe respiratory embarrassment or circulatory collapse is with a 14G i.v. cannula inserted anteriorly through the second intercostal space. More formal drainage is by wide-bore chest drain tube inserted with a sterile technique. Insertion should be under direct vision after dissection down to the pleura. Most physicians recommend inserting the tube in the mid-axillary line at the level of the nipple. The tube should be directed posteriorly especially in the presence of a haemothorax.

- The classic signs of cardiac tamponade include a falling BP and a rising JVP but these signs may be mimicked by a tension pneumothorax. Aspiration of as little as 30 ml pericardial fluid via a xiphisternal approach may produce considerable (but short lived) improvements in haemodynamics. Further surgical definitive care will be necessary.

Penetrating chest injuries

Penetrating chest injuries *all* require surgery, preferably in a specialist centre. However, penetrating cardiac injuries do not normally tolerate the delays associated with interhospital transfer. Emergency room thoracotomy for penetrating cardiac injuries carries a surprisingly good prognosis.[18]

Massive haemothorax

Immediate thoracotomy is indicated according to many chest surgeons if the initial bleed is >1500 ml on insertion of the chest drain or if there is continual drainage after insertion of the chest drain. In theory (and usually in practice) re-expansion of the lung following drainage 'tamponades' the bleeding.

Pain relief

Adequate pain relief is a crucial part of treatment of patients with chest injuries. Acutely, i.v. narcotics should be titrated according to effect. Later there are many suitable techniques largely chosen according to individual preference:

- PCA;
- i.v. infusion of narcotics;
- thoracic epidural is probably the regional anaesthetic technique of choice and has been shown, for example, to be superior to intrapleural catheter;[19]
- non-steriodal anti-inflammatory drugs (NSAIDS) are useful adjuncts especially for simple rib fractures.

Reconsider IPPV

- After acute resuscitation one may have to reconsider the necessity for ventilation.
- In general, this will be dependant on the degree of pulmonary contusion or collapse and the increased work of breathing.

- The overall condition of the patient also has an influence, e.g. a low threshold for IPPV in the presence of other injuries especially head injury, pre-existing chest disease or the elderly patient.

Myocardial contusion

Unexpected arrhythmias are often a clue to the presence of myocardial contusion. Electrocardiogram (ECG) and cardiac enzyme changes are variable and may mimic a myocardial infarction (MI). Treatment is syptomatic and recovery is common unless gross cardiac failure is present.

Pulmonary contusion

- There may be few signs and symptoms in the early period after injury. In addition, an initial CXR may also be normal.

- However, bruised lung like any other bruised tissue becomes more oedematous with time, i.e. pulmonary function will deteriorate over 48 h and IPPV may become necessary.

- 'Avoid over hydration' is good advice but the choice of fluid and the end points of fluid therapy are difficult and controversial.

- There is a high incidence of associated injury especially head and abdominal injuries.

Rib fractures

- There is no specific treatment for rib fractures.

- One should note, however, that first rib fractures are especially serious due to the large force required to cause them to fracture. Thus, there is a high incidence of associated injuries especially mediastinal and brachial plexus injuries.

- Similarly, lower rib fractures are associated with a high incidence of liver and spleen injuries depending on the side fractures are on.

- Elderly rib cages have usually lost their elastic recoil and therefore even injuries with low kinetic energy cause significant fractures. Conversely, the rib cages of the young patient transmit the kinetic energy more readily and can result in significant life-threatening contusion in the absence of rib fractures.

Flail chest

- Flail chest is a functional diagnosis and not a radiological diagnosis.

- The physiological effects are due to four main problems:

  - underlying contusion;

  - impaired elastic recoil leading to pulmonary collapse;

  - increased work of breathing;

  - pain leading to sputum retention.

- The approach varies according to the severity of the chest injury, the severity of associated injuries and the effectiveness of pain relief.

- The best single guide to the requirement for IPPV is the degree of pulmonary contusion.[20]

- Management is either conservative or invasive.

Conservative

- Includes oxygen therapy, adequate analgesia, especially epidural analgesia, and physiotherapy.

- Is indicated in an isolated injury with adequate gas exchange and a good cough.

- Prophylactic IPPV for such patients may increase complications and prolong hospital stay.

Invasive

- The presence of significant contusion, pre-existing chest disease, other significant injuries or an ineffective cough are indications for IPPV.

- Up to 69% of patients with flail chest require mechanical ventilation for an average of 22 days.[21]

- Surgical fixation of the flail segment in the absence of any other indications for thoracotomy is controversial and unproved.

Outcome after multiple injury

- Patients admitted to ICU following multiple injuries often have a protracted length of stay, duration of IPPV and consume a lot of resources.[22]

- Isolated pulmonary contusion in young trauma patients has a good prognosis.[23]

- Length of stay and mortality are increased in the elderly trauma patient with a greater proportion requiring chronic care following discharge from ICU.

- Development of sepsis and multiple organ failure is responsible for much of the late mortality.

- Young trauma patients have a better prognosis and for those who survive they have a good prospect of rehabilitation and a fairly good ultimate outcome.

Further reading

Nolan JP, Parr MJA. Aspects of resuscitation in trauma. *Br J Anaesth* 1997: **79**; 226–40.

Santora TA, Schinco MA, Trooskin SZ. Management of trauma in the elderly patient. *Surg Clin North Am* 1994: **74**; 163–86.

Moore FA, Moore EE. Evolving concepts in the pathogenesis of postinjury multiple organ failure. *Surg Clin North Am* 1995: **75**; 257–77.

Falk JL, O'Brien JF, Kerr R. Fluid resuscitation in traumatic hemorrhagic shock. *Crit Care Clin* 1992: **8**; 323–40.

References

1. Loes O, Smith Erichsen N, Lind B. Intensive care: cost and benefit. *Acta Anaesthesiol Scand* 1987: **31 (suppl.)**; 84–9.

2. Little RA. 1988 Fitts Lecture: Heart rate changes after haemorrhage and injury – a reappraisal. *J Trauma* 1989: **29**; 903–6.

3. Wilmore DW. The wound as an organ. In Little RA, Frayn KN (eds), *The Scientific Basis for the Care of the Critically Ill*. Manchester University Press, 1986.

4. Weil MH, Shubin H. The 'VIP' approach to the bedside management of shock. *JAMA* 1969: **207**; 337–40.

5. Wood PR, Lawler PG. Managing the airway in cervical spine injury. A review of the Advanced Trauma Life Support protocol. *Anaesthesia* 1992: **47**; 792–7.

6. Bickell WH, Wall MJ Jr, Pepe PE *et al*. Immediate versus delayed fluid resuscitation for hypotensive patients with penetrating torso injuries. *N Engl J Med* 1994: **331**; 1105–9.

7. Scalea TM, Simon HM, Duncan AO *et al*. Geriatric blunt multiple trauma: improved survival with early invasive monitoring. *J Trauma* 1990: **30**; 129–34.

8. Abou-Khalil B, Scalea TM, Trooskin SZ *et al*. Hemodynamic responses to shock in young trauma patients: need for invasive monitoring. *Crit Care Med* 1994: **22**; 633–9.

9. Wo CC, Shoemaker WC, Appel PL *et al*. Unreliability of blood pressure and heart rate to evaluate cardiac output in emergency resuscitation and critical illness. *Crit Care Med* 1993: **21**; 218–23.

10. Rutherford EJ, Morris JA Jr, Reed GW, Hall KS. Base deficit stratifies mortality and determines therapy. *J Trauma* 1992: **33**; 417–23.

11. Waisman Y, Eichacker PQ, Banks SM *et al*. Acute hemorrhage in dogs: construction and validation of models to quantify blood loss. *J Appl Physiol* 1993: **74**; 510–19.

12. Bishop MH, Shoemaker WC, Appel PL *et al*. Relationship between supranormal circulatory values, time delays, and outcome in severely traumatized patients. *Crit Care Med* 1993: **21**; 56–63.

13. Bishop MH, Shoemaker WC, Appel PL *et al*. Prospective, randomized trial of survivor values of cardiac index, oxygen delivery, and oxygen consumption as resuscitation endpoints in severe trauma. *J Trauma* 1995: **38**; 780–7.

14. Durham R, Neunaber K, Mazuski J *et al*. The use of oxygen consumption and delivery as endpoints for resuscitation in critically ill patients. *J Trauma* 1996: **41**; 32–40.

15. Ivatury RR, Simon RJ, Havriliak D *et al*. Gastric mucosal pH and oxygen delivery and oxygen consumption indices in the assessment of adequacy of resuscitation after trauma: a prospective, randomized study. *J Trauma* 1995: **39**; 128–34.

16. Johnson KD, Cadambi A, Seibert GB. Incidence of adult respiratory distress syndrome in patients with multiple musculoskeletal injuries: effect of early operative stabilization of fractures. *J Trauma* 1985: **25**; 375–84.

17. Hirshberg A, Mattox KL. 'Damage control' in trauma surgery. *Br J Surg* 1993: **80**; 1501–2.

18. Arreola-Risa C, Rhee P, Boyle EM *et al*. Factors influencing outcome in stab wounds of the heart. *Am J Surg* 1995: **169**; 553–6.

19. Luchette FA, Radafshar SM, Kaiser R *et al*. Prospective evaluation of epidural versus intrapleural catheters for analgesia in chest wall trauma. *J Trauma* 1994: **36**: 865–9.

20. Ciraulo DL, Elliott D, Mitchell KA, Rodriguez A. Flail chest as a marker for significant injuries. *J Am Coll Surg* 1994: **178**; 466–70.

21. Wisner DH A stepwise logistic regression analysis of factors affecting morbidity and mortality after thoracic trauma: effect of epidural analgesia. *J Trauma* 1990: **30**; 799–804.

22. Goins WA, Reynolds HN, Nyanjom D, Dunham CM. Outcome following prolonged intensive care unit stay in multiple trauma patients. *Crit Care Med* 1991: **19**; 339–45.

23. Hoff SJ, Shotts SD, Eddy VA, Morris JA Jr. Outcome of isolated pulmonary contusion in blunt trauma patients. *Ann Surg* 1994: **60**; 138–42.

14

THE PATIENT WITH CARDIAC DYSFUNCTION

D. Roberts

The common cardiac problems in ICU patients are cardiac failure, cardiogenic shock and arrhythmias. As many ICUs also admit 'coronary care' patients, a general overview of management of acute myocardial infarction is presented.

Myocardial infarction MI

- Acute MI remains one of the most common causes of death in Western countries.

- The usual aetiology is occlusive thrombus superimposed on a ruptured or ulcerated coronary atheromatous plaque. The plaques most likely to rupture are those rich in extra cellular lipid covered by a thin fibrous cap and are not necessarily the most severely stenotic lesions.

- Death of cardiac myocytes occurs with prolonged ischaemia due to coronary occlusion, the rate of which is dependent on factors effecting myocardial demands such as heart rate, blood pressure, myocardial contractility and ischaemic preconditioning.

- The formation of an acute coronary thrombus is not a static process but a dynamic one as the artery opens and closes.

- MI usually affects the left ventricle (LV) and intraventricular septum but may affect the right ventricle (60% of patients with inferior MI) or the atria.

- Large MI and anterior MI dilate more than inferior MI with less dilatation and scarring (remodelling) if the infarct-related artery is patent.

Presentation

Typically with retrosternal chest discomfort. Elderly patients or those with diabetes mellitus are more likely to present with atypical symptoms such as heart failure or a stroke. The most important differential diagnosis to consider is aortic dissection (check all pulses!).

Diagnosis

Electrocardiogram (ECG)   The initial one may be normal and if history suggests MI serial ECGs should be performed (every 15–30 min), looking for convex ST segment elevation over the site of infarction (septal, VI–V2; anterior, V3–V4; lateral I, AVL, V5, V6; inferior II, III, AVF; right ventricular involvement, V4R, V3R). MI cannot be reliably diagnosed if left bundle branch block (LBBB) is present.

Cardiac enzymes

- Creatinine kinase (CK) is the most useful enzyme. An increase in CK is seen within 4 h after onset of symptoms, decreasing to normal levels at 48 h. Measurement of isoenzyme CKMB is required for patients who have had cardiopulmonary resuscitation, cardiac surgery or intramuscular injections.

- Aspartate transaminase (AST) is non-specific and rises later after symptom onset (8–12 h) than CK. It is now used less often.

- Lactic dehydrogenase (LDH) is only of use in diagnosis of MI in the patient presenting several days after onset. It is also non-specific and isoenzymes may be required.

- Troponin T can be detected as elevated <4 h after onset of MI and is very sensitive. It is also present for up to 120 h after MI and, thus, is useful for late presenters. There is only minor cross reactivity between myocardial and skeletal troponin T.

Management

- Relief of pain and anxiety. Morphine (with metoclopramide or prochlorperazine to prevent nausea or vomiting).

- Aspirin. All patients without contraindications should receive 75–150 mg immediately and this should be continued long-term, will reduce the mortality rate by 10–15% and the chances of reinfarction by 20–30%.[1,2]

- Thrombolytic therapy. All patients without contraindications who have prolonged ischaemic chest pain and/or new onset ST elevation in two or more leads (>2 mm VI–3, 1 mm in other leads) or new LBBB presenting <12 h after symptom onset should receive this treatment. Patients with ST-segment depression should not be treated as most have non-occlusive thrombi and there is currently no evidence of benefit from thrombolysis. The aim of thrombolysis is to achieve patency of the infarct-related artery as soon as possible. Patency preserves LV function and is associated with a lower mortality rate. Assessment of the safety and risks of thrombolytic therapy is very important.

Thrombolytic agents

- The choice depends on the characteristics of the patient being treated, the safety profile of the agent and cost.

- The most commonly used agents are streptokinase (SK) or recombinant tissue plasminogen activator (RT-PA):

- SK combines with circulating plasminogen to form an activator complex and this converts both circulating plasma and thrombus-bound plasminogen to plasmin. Plasmin lyses fibrin within the thrombus, producing fibrin-degradation products. Activated plasmin also can degrade circulating coagulation proteins, especially fibrinogen. The recommended dose is 1.5 million IU infused over 60 min.

- RT-PA is produced by recombinant DNA technology and has the major advantage of being non-allergenic. It has a much shorter half life than SK. In the GUSTO Trial[3] patients aged between 55 and 75 years and those with anterior MI were shown to have a greater net clinical benefit with 'accelerated' RT-PA (over 90 min) than with SK. RT-PA is expensive and a major indication for its use is in patients who require repeat thrombolysis, having previously received SK (which is antigenic resulting in the development of neutralizing antibodies).

Adverse affects of thrombolytic agents

- Minor bleeding.

- Major bleeding (requires discontinuation of thrombolytic agent, administration of fresh frozen plasma to replenish clotting factors and fibrinogen).

- Hypotension (usually responds to slowing infusion or stopping for 10 min, elevation of legs and i.v. fluid may be necessary).

- Allergy (fever, nausea, skin rash, etc.) can occur. Intravenous antihistamines and hydrocortisone may help. Intravenous adrenaline may be required for a severe reaction.

- Re-perfusion arrhythmias. Other than ventricular fibrillation they are brief and usually revert spontaneously, e.g. idioventricular rhythm.

Adjunctive heparin therapy

Administration of SK or RT-PA is associated with activation of thrombin, which is thrombogenic. Heparin blocks thrombin in plasma but is relatively ineffective against clot-bound thrombin. Theoretically, this appears beneficial after thrombolysis with both RT-PA and SK, by improving initial patency and preventing reocclusion. However, no study has shown benefit over aspirin alone and firm recommendations regarding heparin cannot be made at present.

Percutaneous transluminal coronary angioplasty (PTCA)

PTCA can be used in different ways to treat patients with acute MI.

- Primary PTCA is performed in patients without prior administration of thrombolysis. In some centres this approach may be better than thrombolysis as far as mortality reduction and rate of reinfarction are concerned.[4] However, it is costly and requires a dedicated team and immediate access to a cardiac catheter laboratory 24 h a day. It has a clear role however, in patients with major contraindications to thrombolysis such as a history of recent stroke, uncontrolled hypertension, proliferative diabetic retinopathy, recent surgery, a recent peptic ulcer or a bleeding disorder. It may also be particularly useful for patients early in cardiogenic shock (within the first 24 h).[5]

- PTCA can also be performed in patients with symptoms of recurrent myocardial ischaemia after thrombolysis, which is refractory to medical therapy. It can also be used in patients who fail to re-perfuse following thrombolysis, e.g. when ST segments remain elevated.

β-Blockers

β-Adrenoceptor blocking agents inhibit the arrhythmogenic effect of catecholamines and reduce myocardial demands by affecting heart rate, blood pressure and contractility. A number of trials have shown that i.v. administration reduces hospital mortality and morbidity rates by 15% and also reduces the incidence of ventricular fibrillation and reinfarction.[6] In the first international study of infarct survival (ISIS-1)[7] the major benefit of i.v. atenolol was a reduced incidence of myocardial rupture.[8] The precise role of β-blockers adjunctive to thrombolytic therapy is not clearly defined. They are strongly recommended for MI patients (without contraindications to β-blockade) who do not receive thrombolytic therapy.

Angiotensin converting enzyme (ACE) inhibitors

Pooled results of recent trials have shown than administration of ACE inhibitors on day 1 after acute MI reduces the mortality rate by 6.5%. These trials include the CONSENSUS-2 Trial[9] with enalapril and the GISSI-3 Study[10] using lisinopril. Patients with anterior MI, previous MI or heart failure benefited most. Oral therapy (test dose initially) should begin 2 h after thrombolysis (or β-blockade) if systolic blood pressure >100 mmHg, and should be continued long-term.

Non-invasive assessment of LV function (usually by echocardiography) should be performed prior to hospital discharge in all other MI patients and, in those with impaired contractility (ejection fraction <40%, including those with inferior MI), ACE inhibitor therapy should be initiated.

Nitrates (see also Heart failure, page 137)

Intravenous nitroglycerin is very useful for recurrent ischaemia following MI and there may be a small survival benefit with its use. It dilates the epicardial coronary arteries and increases collateral blood flow. Nitrate therapy is also beneficial for the management of pulmonary oedema by dilating the pulmonary veins, decreasing LV preload and myocardial oxygen demands. The infusion should be started at 5–10 mcg/min and increased every 5–10 min according to clinical response and blood pressure. However, patients on prolonged infusion may develop tolerance. Nitrate therapy should only be given with extreme caution to patients with right ventricular involvement associated with MI in case filling pressure falls dramatically.

Arrhythmia prophylaxis

Many ventricular arrhythmias following MI are relatively benign or self limiting. The dangers of overzealous attempts at arrhythmia prophylaxis were illustrated by the CAST study (Cardiac Arrhythmia Suppression Trial) in which use of Flecainide and Encainide in MI patients to suppress ventricular ectopics resulted in a higher mortality rate than when using the placebo.[11] Routine prophylaxis with lignocaine is also no longer recommended.[12]

Cardiogenic shock

This is usually caused by acute MI and is characterized by:

- Pallor.
- Systolic blood pressure <90 mmHg.
- Cold, clammy extremities.
- Oliguria (<20ml/h).
- Cerebral hypoperfusion (presenting as confusion, etc.).
- CI <1.8 l/min/m^2.
- High pulmonary capillary wedge pressure (PCWP).

Management

- Mortality is high as may be associated with loss of >40% of the LV.
- It is important to treat precipitating causes or exacerbating factors such as an arrhythmia or severe hypoxia.

- Measurement of PCWP and cardiac output using a pulmonary artery catheter is usually indicated.

- The PCWP will be high but care must be taken not to allow this to fall too low in response to treatment.

- Reduction of afterload is also desirable but systemic hypotension may preclude the use of nitrate infusions and inotropic support is often necessary in such circumstances.

- Uncontrolled studies suggest that PTCA may improve the survival in cardiogenic shock.[5]

Intra-aortic balloon pumping (IABP)

Useful for stabilizing shocked patients with surgically correctable complications (e.g. ventricular septal defect following MI) and also those with potentially viable myocardium ('myocardial stunning'), e.g. following PTCA. The balloon is introduced percutaneously via the femoral artery into the aorta. Synchronized with the cardiac cycle, the IABP is inflated during diastole to augment pressure in the proximal aorta and thus to improve coronary filling. The deflation during systole also effectively reduces tension in the aorta and reduces the impedance to LV ejection or afterload. The resultant effects of the IABP are to increase cardiac output (CO) and reduce PCWP.

Right ventricular infarction

- Patients with right ventricular (RV) infarction usually have an elevated jugular venous pressure (JVP) that does not fall in inspiration (Kussmaul's sign) and may develop hypotension and peripheral vasoconstriction without pulmonary congestion.

- Diagnosis can be confirmed by performing right-sided chest lead measurement on the ECG (elevated ST segment in V3R or V4R), echocardiography or nuclear imaging (if available).

- Invasive monitoring shows the CVP to be elevated out of proportion to the PCWP. The PCWP may indeed be normal or even low.

- Major haemodynamic disturbances may occur and rapid infusion of fluid volume can produce immediate improvement by raising LV end diastolic pressure (LVEDP) and CO.

- Caution may need to be exercised as overzealous fluid loading can cause dilation of the RV with further falls in RV ejection. Dobutamine or dopamine may therefore be required to 'support' the RV if volume expansion alone is not sufficient.

- Patients with RV infarction who require pacing (temporary or permanent) benefit haemodynamically from right atrioventricular sequential (DDD) pacing rather than just ventricular (VVI) pacing.

- The prognosis after RV infarction is usually good with appropriate treatment as spontaneous improvement in RV function occurs over several days. The long-term prognosis is dependent on LV involvement.

Heart failure

Heart failure occurs when a myocardial abnormality causes CO to fail to meet the body's demands. 'High output' failure, in contrast, occurs when CO is excessively increased due, for example, to anaemia, thyrotoxicosis, Paget's disease, etc. The high output state may also exacerbate or bring out an underlying myocardial problem (e.g. previously asymptomatic coronary artery disease). Heart failure may be due to *systolic* (inability of the muscle to shorten, e.g. secondary to coronary artery disease) or *diastolic* dysfunction (when the myocardium is slow to relax due to increased chamber stiffness, e.g. from hypertension or again from coronary heart disease).

With the development of heart failure neurohumoral changes occur, e.g. activation of the sympathetic nervous and renin–angiotensin systems. In the severely compromised patient a vicious cycle occurs with peripheral vasoconstriction (increased 'afterload'), decreasing CO, tachycardia (increasing myocardial oxygen demands) and raised LV filling pressures (increased 'preload') decreasing subendocardial perfusion.

The diverse aetiology and poor prognosis of established heart failure makes precise diagnosis essential for correct treatment (Table 1). Equally the precipitating cause, e.g. a cardiac arrhythmia, leading to presentation should be sought and treated (Table 2). Investigation is aimed mainly at:

- confirming the presence of LV dysfunction (usually by echocardiography);

- excluding operable valve disease;

- detecting coronary artery disease where surgery would be appropriate;

- obtaining prognostic information.

Management of severe heart failure

Immediate management

- Conscious patients are usually more comfortable sitting up.

- High flow oxygen therapy (see the chapter on Oxygen therapy).

Table 14.1 – Causes of heart failure.

Direct myocardial damage
- Coronary artery disease
- Cardiomyopathy
- Myocarditis
- Alcohol

Volume overload, e.g.:
- Aortic or mitral regurgitation
- Post-infarction ventricular septal defect

Pressure Overload, e.g.:
- Aortic stenosis
- Hypertension

Impaired ventricular filling, e.g.:
- Mitral stenosis
- Hypertrophic cardiomyopathy

Table 14.2 – Precipitating cause of heart failure.

Arrhythmias, especially atrial fibrillation with a rapid ventricular rate
Infection, especially pneumonia in the elderly
Anaemia, again more frequent in the elderly
Infective endocarditis
Thyrotoxicosis
Drug therapy, e.g. non-steroidal anti-inflammatory agents

- Diamorphine 2.5–5 mg i.v. plus an antiemetic drug.

  Frusemide 40–80 mg i.v. or bumetanide 1–2 mg i.v. This produces immediate benefit from vasodilatation, then diuresis in 5–30 min.

- Investigations, i.e. ECG, CXR, routine blood tests. An echocardiogram is urgently required if mechanical causes are suspected.

Management strategies

Diuretics   Diuretics enhance renal sodium and water excretion and in acute failure can also reduce ventricular filling pressure (possibly mediated through prostaglandin activation). In practice, three classes of diuretics are used:

- loop diuretics (frusemide or bumetanide) that act at the loop of Henlé;

- thiazides, which act at the cortical diluting segment;

- potassium-sparing agents (e.g. spironolactone, amiloride) that act in the distal tubule.

Watch for hypokalaemia and/or hyponatraemia.

Vasodilators

Nitrates   (see also MI). Nitrates are especially useful when failure is due to underlying ischaemia and/or mitral regurgitation. They can be administered orally, by the buccal or sublingual routes, topically or i.v.. Intravenous therapy can be isosorbide dinitrate 2–10 mg/h or glyceryl trinitrate 10–200 mcg/min with careful monitoring of systolic blood pressure (try and maintain >90 mmHg).

Sublingual nitrate in the emergency room can have a rapidly beneficial effect.[13]

ACE inhibitors   There are many different actions of ACE inhibitors, but the primary effect is to attenuate the increased production of angiotensin II. This leads to a reduced plasma concentration of aldosterone and arginine vasopressin (AVP), decreased sympathetic activity plus increased parasympathetic activity. Both arterial and venous dilatation occur, principally as a result of inhibition of circulating (and possibly tissue) ACE. Both cardiac filling pressures and myocardial wall stress are reduced and cardiac output may increase. Life expectancy is extended in all grades of heart failure[14,15] and asymptomatic LV dysfunction, while symptoms such as dyspnoea and exercise capacity improve.

Adverse affects include:

- hypotension (including 'first dose' effect);
- renal impairment (regular monitoring essential);
- cough (5% of patients);
- skin rashes.

Hypotension occurs most often in dehydrated patients or in those receiving excessive diuretics. In severe heart failure with low systolic blood pressure (<90 mmHg) the dose should be titrated cautiously using the short-acting agents such as captopril starting at 6.25 mg bd or even 1 mg bd.

Orally active angiotensin 11 antagonists are also being studied for the treatment of heart failure (and hypertension). Losartan is specific for the subtype 1 (AT1) receptor (which regulates blood pressure and aldosterone secretion) and may be useful in patients who are intolerant to ACE inhibitors.

β-Adrenoceptor agonists   Dopamine and dobutamine are sympathomimetic amines administered i.v. with positive inotropic actions. For these drugs and their use, see Chapter 8. ECG monitoring is essential with these drugs as they can be arrhythmogenic.

β-Adrenoceptor antagonists   The role of β-blockers in chronic heart failure is controversial and the mechanism of any benefit is also unclear. New agents, e.g. with other vasoactive properties, such as carvedilol, show most promise.

Digoxin Digoxin has complex direct and indirect electrophysiological effects (see the section on arrhythmias) and is the drug of first choice to control the ventricular rate in patients with atrial fibrillation (restoration of sinus rhythm may be a better option by electrical or pharmacological cardioversion, however). There has been much debate on the role of digoxin in patients with heart failure who remain in sinus rhythm. Its inotropic effect is mild but it may inhibit the sympathetic nervous system in heart failure leading to arterial vasodilation. It is of little use in acute heart failure but may have a role in chronic heart failure unresponsive to other treatments.

IPPV and cardiac failure

As discussed in Chapter 6, the effects of IPPV on cardiac function are complex and differ according to the underlying state of the heart. The best evidence for a clinically beneficial effect of IPPV in heart failure is indirect, i.e. deterioration of cardiac function during weaning from IPPV. However, there is additional evidence for significant, beneficial effects of ventilatory support in heart failure:

- Oxygenation is improved.

- Pulmonary oedema may be improved:

    - alveolar fluid partially redistributed to the interstitial space further improving oxygenation;

    - prevention of oedema formation;

    - prevention of alveolar collapse in the dependant portion of the lung secondary to the 'weight' of the fluid filled lung.

- In animal studies of cardiogenic shock, respiratory arrest is usually the mode of death due to diaphragmatic fatigue secondary to increased work of breathing. IPPV will eliminate the increased work of breathing.

- Face mask CPAP may be beneficial in cardiac failure and cardiogenic shock.[16]

- High-frequency jet ventilation synchronized with the cardiac cycle can increase intrathoracic pressure only during systole, reducing LV afterload while avoiding the reductions in preload during diastole. Early results with this technique show improvements in cardiac output and oxygenation.[17]

Cardiac transplantation

Heart transplantation is still the only option for patients who have minimal LV function. Although a palliative procedure the benefits are enormous with >80% alive at 1 year and 60% alive at 5 years with an improved quality of life. Suitable, generally young, patients should be discussed with a cardiologist once the patients are out of ICU or off the ventilator.

Cardiac arrhythmias and their management

Arrhythmias are very common in ICU patients – a general prevalence of 78% in one study of 2820 patients.[18] Atrial fibrillation is the commonest serious arrhythmia in the critically ill patient, occurring in 52 % of ICU patients at some point in their illness.

Tachycardias with narrow ventricular complexes

Atrial fibrillation (AF)   In established AF, drug therapy is usually used to control the rate of ventricular response by increasing atrioventricular nodal refractoriness. Vagal manoeuvres will do this temporarily and may be useful in the diagnosis of fast AF. Digoxin is still the drug of choice, however. If the ventricular response is still too fast in a well-digitalized patient, low-dose β-blockade or verapamil (check LV function) can be added. If this fails amiodarone can be tried.

- In paroxysmal AF, therapy is aimed at reducing the frequency of arrhythmia attacks and amiodarone, sotalol or flecainide (the latter two only if LV function is preserved) are the most effective agents.

- DC cardioversion should be considered for an 'attack of AF' or where atrial transport is vital to the maintenance of a reasonable cardiac output (e.g. in patients with poor LV function). Prior anticoagulation should always be considered.

- AF can also be chemically cardioverted into sinus rhythm using amiodarone, procainamide, disopyramide or flecainide. Amiodarone is the drug of choice in patients with impaired LV function.

- Magnesium deficiency is common in critically ill patients. Magnesium sulphate is effective in many ICU patients for controlling the rate in AF or even converting AF back to sinus rhythm.

- In critically ill patients, AF can be precipitated by hypovolaemia and respond to fluid therapy.[19]

Atrial flutter   The atrial rate in atrial flutter is 280–320/min and 2:1 ventricular response results in a ventricular rate of 150/min. Carotid sinus massage (CSM) will increase the degree of atrioventricular block temporarily and this be useful in diagnosis as the 'saw-tooth' pattern of atrial flutter becomes obvious. An isolated event is best treated by DC cardioversion. Paroxsymal atrial flutter responds to digoxin (AF may be produced) while amiodarone may be useful in reducing rapid ventricular rates.

Atrial or supra ventricular tachycardia (SVT)   The atrial rate is 150–250/min and the ventricular response is frequently 1:1. P waves may not be visible on the ECG but often appear with carotid sinus massage. Adenosine (3–6 mg rapid i.v. followed by 12 mg after 1–2 min if necessary) or verapamil (1–10 mg i.v. over 5 min) are the drugs of choice in an acute episode.

Junctional tachycardia   This is usually due to re-entry within the atrioventricular node. Accessory extra-nodal pathways, e.g. Wolff–Parkinson–White syndrome, may be involved in the circuit. AV nodal blocking drugs, e.g. verapamil, β-blockade or adenosine, are usually effective.

Tachycardias with broad ventricular complexes

These can be due to:

- ventricular tachycardia (VT);

- SVT when bundle branch block has already been present during sinus rhythm;

- SVT with rate-related bundle branch block.

Pointers towards VT include:

- presence of myocardial damage;

- evidence of independent atrial activity;

- QRS duration >0.14 s;

- a concordant ECG pattern, i.e. all positive or negative in the chest leads (VI–V6);

- marked axis deviation;

- capture/fusion beats.

Always try to obtain a 12-lead ECG during tachycardia and compare this with the patient's 12-lead ECG during sinus rhythm wherever possible.

Management of VT

Treatment of VT depends on the patient's condition:

- Blood should be checked for potassium, acid–base balance and blood gases, and a correction made if necessary.

- In the sick patient with a low output state, cardiac massage may be required and immediate DC cardioversion is necessary.

Table 14.3 – Drugs used to treat cardiac arrythmias.

Drug	Vaughan–Williams class	Intravenous dose	Oral dose
Quinidine	Ia	Very rarely used	600/1200 mg in divided doses (rarely used)
Procainamide	Ia	100 mg over 5 min + 2–5 mg/min as infusion	375 mg 4 hourly (rarely used but valuable in 'resistant' VT)
Disopyramide	Ia	50 mg over 5 min (max 300 mg in 1 h)	100–200 mg QDS
Lignocaine	Ib	100–200 mg i.v. bolus + 1–4 mg/min	not applicable
Mexiletine	Ib	100–250 mg over 10 min 4 mg/min for 1 h then 2 mg/min for 1 h then 0.5 mg/min	200 mg TDS
Phenytoin	Ib	10–15 mg/kg over 1 h	400–600 mg daily
Flecainide	Ic	1.5–2 mg/kg over 10 min	100–200 mg bd
Propafenone	Ic	not applicable	150–300 mg tds
Propanolol	II	0.1–0.2 mg/kg over 5 min	40 mg tds (range 10–240 mg tds)
Amiodarone*	III	5 mg/kg over 2–4 h + 10–20 mg/kg/day (1–2 days)	200 mg tds for 1 week reducing to 200 mg od or less
Sotalol	III	20–60 mg over 2–3 min	120–640 mg daily in single/divided doses
Bretylium Tosylate (very useful for resistant VT)	III	5–10 mg/kg over 10 min then 1–2 mg/min	not applicable
Verapamil	IV	5–10 mg over 2 min	80–120 mg tds; 240–480 mg daily of slow release preparation (caution in combination with β-blocker)
Adenosine	V	rapid 6 mg bolus; 12 mg bolus may be given once more after 2min	not applicable

All antiarrhythmic drugs have proarrhythmic effects (especially watch the QT interval and for evidence of 'torsade de pointes'). In addition, caution should be exerted in patients with conduction abnormalities on the resting ECG in sinus rhythm and further caution should be exerted in patients with LV dysfunction/hypotension.
*Drugs safer with impaired LV function.

- If VT is well tolerated, lignocaine 100–200 mg i.v. should be given followed by an infusion (4 mg/min for 30 min, 2 mg/min for 2 h, then 1 mg/min).

- If lignocaine fails to control the VT alternative drugs are tried, preferably from different classes in the Vaughan–Williams Classification (table 3).

- 'Overdrive' right ventricular pacing may also occasionally be useful in resistant cases.

- Once successfully cardioverted, prophylactic therapy is started orally. The effect of the chosen drug is monitored with telemetry and/or Holter monitoring.

- It is important to keep the serum potassium between 4.5 and 5.5 mmol/l and to exclude hypomagnesaemia (especially in patients already on diuretics).

- If VT were secondary to MI or acute myocarditis antiarrhythmic, therapy should probably only be continued for 3 months in the first instance. Repeat Holter monitoring on drug therapy and after its withdrawal is advised.

In some cases more than one drug will be necessary and indefinite oral therapy may be required. Alternatively an implantable cardioverter/defibrillator should be considered.

Further reading

Califf RM, Bengtson JR. Cardiogenic shock. *N Engl J Med* 1994;**330**: 1724–30.

Lieu TA, Gurley RJ, Lundstrom RJ, Parmley WW. Primary angioplasty and thrombolysis for acute myocardial infarction: an evidence summary. *J Am Coll Cardiol* 1996; **27**: 737–50.

American College of Cardiology, American Heart Association Task Force Report: Guidelines for the evaluation and management of heart failure. *Circulation* 1995; **92**: 2764–84.

Ahmed R, Singh BN, Antiarrhythmic drugs. *Curr Opinion Cardiol* 1994; **8**: 10–21.

References

1. ISIS-2 (Second International Study of Infant Survival) Collaborative Group. Randomised trial of intravenous streptokinase, oral aspirin, both, or neither among 17 187 cases of suspected acute myocardial infarction: ISIS-2. *Lancet* 1988; **ii**: 349–60.

2. Antiplatelet Trialists' Collaboration. Secondary prevention of vascular disease by prolonged antiplatelet treatment. *BMJ* 1988; **296**: 320–31.

3. The GUSTO Angiographic Investigators. The effects of tissue plasminogen activator, streptokinase, or both on coronary-artery patency, ventricular function, and survival after acute myocardial infarction. *N Engl J Med* 1993; **329**: 1615–22.

4. Grimes CL, Browne KF, Marco J. A comparison of immediate angioplasty with thrombolytic therapy for acute myocardial infarction. *N Engl J Med* 1993; **328**: 673–9.

5. Hibbard MD, Holmes DR, Bailey KR *et al*. Percutaneous transluminal coronary angioplasty in patients with cardiogenic shock. *J Am Coll Cardiol* 1992; **19**: 639–46.

6. Yasuf S, Peto R, Lewis J *et al*. Beta blockade during and after myocardial infarction: an overview of the randomised trials. *Prog Cardiovasc Dis* 1985; **27**: 335–71.

7. First International Study of infant Survival Collaborative Group. Randomised trial of intravenous atenolol among 16,027 cases of suspected acute myocardial infarction: ISIS-1. *Lancet* 1986; **ii**: 57–66.

8. ISIS-1 Collaborative Group. Mechanisms for the early mortality reduction produced by beta blockade started early in acute myocardial infarction: ISIS-1. *Lancet* 1988; **i**: 921–3.

9. Swedberg K, Held P, Kjekshus J *et al*. Effects of the early administration of enalapril on mortality in patients with acute myocardial infarction: results of the Co-operative New Scandinavian Enalapril Survival Study II (CONSENSUS II). *N Engl J Med* 1992; **327**: 678–84.

10. Gruppo Italiano per lo Studio della Sopravvivenza nell'infarto Miocardico. GISSI-3: effects of lisinopril and transdermal glyceryl trinitrate singly and together on 6-week mortality and ventricular function after acute myocardial infarction. *Lancet* 1994 ; **343**: 1115–22.

11. Echt DS, Liebson PR, Mitchell LB *et al*. Mortality and morbidity in patients receiving encainide, flecainide, or placebo. The Cardiac Arrhythmia Suppression Trial. *N Engl J Med* 1991: **324**: 781–8.

12. Calvin JE, Parrillo JE. Lidocaine and acute coronary care. *Crit Care Med* 1993: **21**: 179–81.

13. Edwards JD, Grant PT, Plunkett P, Nightingale P. The haemodynamic effects of sublingual nitroglycerin spray in severe left ventricular failure. *Int Care Med* 1989:**15**: 247–9.

14. The CONSENSUS Trial Study Group. Effects of enalapril on mortality in severe congestive heart failure. *N Engl J Med* 1987; **316**: 1429–35.

15. The SOLVD Investigators. Effects of enalapril on survival in patients with reduced left ventricular ejection fractions and congestive heart failure. *N Engl J Med* 1991; **325**: 293–302.

16. Bersten AD, Holt AW, Vedig AE *et al*. Treatment of severe cardiogenic pulmonary oedema with continuous positive airway pressure delivered by face mask. *N Engl J Med* 1991: **325**: 1825–30.

17. Pinsky MR, Marquez J, Martin D, Klain M. Ventricular assist by cardiac cycle-specific increases in intrathoracic pressure. *Chest* 1987: **91**: 709–15.

18. Artucio H, Pereira M. Cardiac arrhythmias in critically ill patients: epidemiologic study. *Crit Care Med* 1990: **18**: 1383–8.

19. Edwards JD, Wilkins RG. Atrial fibrillation precipitated by acute hypovolaemia. *BMJ* 1987: **294**: 283–4

15

THE PATIENT WITH SEPSIS

Sepsis, either as the cause of admission or acquired on the ICU, is:

- the leading cause of multiple organ failure;

- the leading cause of ARDS;

- the leading cause of late death in trauma patients;

- probably the commonest cause of renal failure in surgical patients;

- there are an estimated 300,000 cases of Gram-negative sepsis each year in the USA;

- an estimated 40,000 of these will go on to develop septic shock;

- the mortality of septic shock varies in studies from 40 to 80%.

Definitions

There has been poor agreement on the terminology of sepsis, which perhaps explains the wide variation of reported mortality rates in old studies on septic shock. (For example, 'septic shock' which responds well to fluid loading would not surprisingly have a better prognosis than if inotropes and vasopressors were required.) Thus it is important that clinicians and researchers use the same definitions. The following terminology has been proposed by a Consensus Conference:[1]

- *Infection*. A host response to the presence of microorganisms or tissue invasion by microorganisms.

- *Bacteraemia*. Defined as the presence of viable bacteria in circulating blood.

- *Sepsis*. A systemic response to infection. Defined[1] as infection plus two or more of:

- temperature >38 or <36°C;

- heart rate >90 beats/min;

- respiratory rate >20 breaths/min or pCO_2 <4.3 kPa;

- WCC >12,000 or >10% immature band forms.

- *Systemic inflammatory response syndrome (SIRS)*. Two or more of the above features of sepsis but in the absence of an infective cause. This recognizes that certain other pathological conditions can stimulate the body to respond in an identical fashion to that of infection, e.g. trauma, burns, pancreatitis. If SIRS or sepsis proceeds to severe sepsis or septic shock the mortality increases.

- *Severe sepsis*. Sepsis associated with organ dysfunction (e.g. oliguria) or hypotension but not requiring inotropic support or vasopressors.

- *Septic shock*. This refers to the occurrence of shock in the presence of sepsis. This was defined[1] as sepsis with hypotension not responding to fluid therapy and organ dysfunction or evidence of tissue hypoxia, e.g. lactic acidosis.

The terms septicaemia and sepsis syndrome have been abandoned.

SIRS is an important concept. It emphasizes that the host response to infectious and non-infectious stimuli is the same and that the severity of the response determines the outcome. An epidemiological study of SIRS broadly supports this and shows in some patients progression with time from SIRS to septic shock.[2]

- However, it has been suggested that the diagnosis of SIRS can be 'too easy' with one study of trauma patients in the ICU showing that while only 10% of patients did not fulfil the criteria for SIRS, only the development of shock was associated with increased mortality.[3]

Owing to the significance of the development of shock from sespis,[3] it is septic shock that we will mainly be discussing in this chapter.

Pathophysiology: the cytokine cascade

Cytokines[4]

- Cytokines are small proteins produced by many cells especially white blood cells.

- Cytokines are similar to hormones but with certain essential differences, e.g. they act locally as well as systemically, self augment as opposed to negative feedback and their effects outlive their appearance in the circulation.

- There are many cytokines with more being identified all the time. Understanding of the pathways is progressing but so far has not been mirrored by therapeutic advances.

- Although reference is made to a cytokine cascade, this is not a cascade in the usual sense with release of a substance directly causing the release of the next substance and so on (e.g. the coagulation cascade). Rather it is more of a complex network with many inter-relationships and links. This has hampered therapeutic intervention as blocking one link in the network may not affect other links which can 'bypass' the therapeutic blockage of the cascade. Indeed, some cytokines are probably initiators of the pathological pathways, others are perpetrators which cause the harmful effects (both worth inhibiting) while others may be likened to innocent bystanders, i.e. markers of the inflammatory response with no direct pathological actions. Efforts to inhibit their effects would be fruitless.

- Cytokines are endogenous pyrogens and may cause the fever seen in sepsis.

- Nitric oxide, a potent vasodilator, is released from endothelium.

- The intrinsic coagulation and complement systems are activated. Disseminated intravascular coagulation (DIC) can occur.

- One group of cytokines which seem to be involved in the pathogenesis of septic shock include the interleukins, especially IL-1 and IL-6 and tumour necrosis factor (TNF).

- Gram-negative bacteria contain endotoxin. Endotoxin stimulates the release of TNF and initiates the cytokine cascade. Gram-positive bacteria also cause the release of TNF by a less well-understood mechanism.

- Studies have shown that after administration of endotoxin there is a rapid rise (peak levels at 90 min) in TNF followed by rises in IL-1 and later rises in IL-6. IL-6 levels show the greatest rise.

- In addition to pathological interest, cytokines are of interest prognostically with, for example, levels of IL-6 being directly related to mortality.[5]

Cardinal pathophysiological and clinical manifestations of sepsis

Myocardial depression

At first glance it seems a paradox to talk of myocardial depression in a condition frequently associated with a higher than normal cardiac index. However:

- the cardiac index is often partially maintained by tachycardia, i.e. stroke volume is reduced;

- there is depression of left ventricle (LV) ejection fraction (LVEF), LV and right ventricle (RV) dilation once preload is restored.[6] Dilation may be an attempt to maintain stroke volume;

- in survivors the abnormality in LVEF is corrected by 7–10 days.

The decrease in myocardial function is due to:

- a circulating myocardial depressant factor;[7]

- a relative circulatory resistance to catecholamines;

- often, a fall in coronary perfusion pressure;

- in late stages a rise in PVR;

- *in vitro* studies also suggest a direct negative inotropic effect of nitric oxide.[8]

Vasodilation

- Nitric oxide, previously known as endothelium derived relaxing factor (EDRF), is the principal mediator of vascular smooth muscle tone. Its release from vascular endothelium, stimulated by endotoxin and cytokines, is the principal cause of the profound vasodilation seen in sepsis causing the characteristic fall in SVR. Nitric oxide is synthesized from the amino acid, arginine, by the action of nitric oxide synthase.

- The degree of vasodilation or peripheral vascular failure may be a major determinant of mortality.[9] Cardiac output (CO) is generally well maintained, even elevated in response to the peripheral vasodilation.

- In severe cases the vasculature can lose its responsiveness to vasopressors.

Leaky capillaries

- Neutrophils may adhere to the damaged endothelial cells releasing proteases and oxygen free radicals which cause further endothelial damage.

- The endothelial damage results in increased vascular wall permeability which leads to peripheral oedema. The leaky capillaries are *not* an indication for either fluid restriction or diuretics. Diuretics do not treat vascular damage.

Decreased circulating volume

- Leaky capillaries contribute to effective hypovolaemia.

- This is in addition to surgical 'third space losses', fluid and blood loss in surgical sepsis and peritonitis

Hypotension

From a combination of all of the above, hypotension is produced. This would not be so bad in the face of a high flow from the elevated CI if there was not an abnormal maldistribution of flow. For example, renal blood flow is impaired at an early stage.

Oxygen transport

- VO_2 is reduced in septic shock often with evidence of tissue hypoxia, i.e. elevated lactate and decease in pHi,[10] often despite well maintained CO and DO_2. In septic shock this may be due to the maldistribution of blood flow, metabolic abnormalities, endothelial cell swelling or increased cellular membrane permeability.

- The inadequate VO_2 might suggest that DO_2 is inadequate to maintain VO_2 and needs to be increased to achieve 'optimal goals' (see Chapter 1). Some have taken the increase in lactate as evidence for *pathological supply dependency* (i.e. straight-line relationship between DO_2 and VO_2 over a wide range of values) and promoted therapy to increase DO_2 and VO_2. However, as outlined in Chapter 1, more modern studies where DO_2 and VO_2 are measured independently do not support widespread occurrence of oxygen supply dependency.

Metabolic changes

- Endotoxin and other cytokine mediators, especially the interleukins, stimulate metabolic changes including protein catabolism and pancreatic secretion of glucagon and insulin.. This septic stimulus induces a sequential, progressive inability to use glucose, fat then amino acids as energy sources.

- This defect is initially expressed peripherally in the muscles and results in an increase in anaerobic metabolism and gluconeogenesis.

- This peripheral defect if prolonged may result in central organ changes ultimately culminating in multiple organ failure.

- These changes are probably induced by adrenergic stimulation, hormonal changes and direct cytokine effects on cellular function and membrane permeability.

Clinical features of septic shock

Localized:

- Pleuritis.
- Peritonitis.

- Mass/abscess.
- Localized tenderness.

Generalized:

- Tachypnoea.
- Hypotension.
- Altered conscious level.
- Fever.
- Hypothermia.
- Rigors.
- General malaise.

Laboratory signs:

- Increased (or sometimes decreased) WCC.
- Thrombocytopenia (sometimes thrombocythaemic response to chronic sepsis).
- Hypoxaemia.
- Hypocarbia.
- Metabolic acidosis with elevated lactate.
- Specific cultures of microorganisms.
- Endotoxin levels (experimental only).

Classically septic shock has been subdivided into early 'warm' shock and late 'cold' shock with features as follows:

Warm shock:

- Hyperdynamic.
- Warm skin.
- Fever and chills.
- Moderate hypotension.
- Moderate urine output.
- Bounding pulse.
- Tachypnoea.
- Low SVR.

- High cardiac output.
- Classically Gram-negative.

- Cold shock:
  - Hypodynamic.
  - Cold and clammy.
  - Mottled skin.
  - Circulatory collapse.
  - Tachypnoea.
  - Oliguria.
  - Thready pulse.
  - High SVR.
  - Low cardiac output.
  - Classically Gram-positive.
  - However it is now recognized that there is no clear distinction in the clinical or haemodynamic profile of Gram-negative or -positive septic shock, i.e. the clinical features give no reliable clue to the nature of the infective organism.
  - Any microorganisms can cause septic shock including fungi.
  - Although some patients may pass from a 'warm' phase to a cold 'phase' (especially if referral is delayed) it is now recognized that the clinical features can be blurred with up to one-third of patients seemingly presenting with 'cold' shock with no prior hyperdynamic phase.[11]

Diagnosis of septic shock

- The diagnosis of septic shock is made on the above clinical and laboratory features especially in an appropriate setting for sepsis, e.g. following laparotomy.

- Cultures may not identify a causative organism (as few as 50% of patients with septic shock will have positive blood cultures). This should not necessarily reassure one that there is no organism! Positive blood or other cultures are not necessary for the diagnosis to be made.

- A strong index of suspicion is necessary especially in the immunosuppressed or patients on corticosteroids who may not show the usual clinical manifestations.

- In cases of acute collapse there will be no time to wait for the results of specific cultures and empirical therapy including empirical choice of antibiotics is promptly required.

- Septic shock can mimic other conditions. Common sense should alert one to the possibility in an appropriate setting, e.g. following abdominal surgery.

- A common error is to falsely ascribe tachypnoea (a cardinal sign) to heart failure.

Therapy of septic shock

Prevention

- Prevention may be easier than cure.

- Therefore the guidelines in Chapter 9 should be followed.

- Prophylactic antibiotics for certain surgical procedures are appropriate.

- Prompt investigation and treatment of postoperative pyrexia and infection.

Eradicate the infection

- The source of the sepsis must be promptly identified and appropriate antibiotics administered and surgical collections drained.

- Gram-negative bacterial lysis by antibiotics may be associated with a sudden release of endotoxin into the bloodstream ('fuelling the fire'). This should not limit the early administration of antibiotic therapy.

- Intravenous catheters suspected of being colonized or infected must be removed and cultured.

Supportive care

- General measures such as fluid therapy, nutritional support and IPPV must be applied as part of the general care of the critically ill patient.

- Managing the patient with septic shock in an ICU run by trained ICU specialists has been shown to improve survival.[12]

- Antibiotic therapy or cardiovascular support alone will provide disappointing results in the therapy of septic shock. Outcome is, perhaps obviously, improved when both are combined.[13]

Haemodynamic and oxygen transport management

- Preload should be optimized as an initial step. However, it has been shown that some patients with septic shock show a diminished cardiovascular response to fluid loading – evidence for the depressed cardiac function of sepsis. Fluid loading alone is unlikely to restore haemodynamic stability, especially if there is RV compromise.[14] Thus almost all patients will require cardiovascular support.

- Early studies purported to show an improved survival when patients were treated to attain the 'optimal goals' (see Chapter 1) of survivors. Unfortunately these studies were, in general, poorly controlled and non-randomized. More recent studies suggest that over aggressive inotropic support in an attempt to achieve these goals, often in elderly patients, results in a worse outcome.[15] It would seem that it is the spontaneous ability (i.e. the cardiac reserve) of the patients to generate these 'supranormal' cardiovascular values that is important for survival. Thus, it is not disputed that there are survivors' haemodynamic values. What is disputed is that one can improve survival in other patients by achieving these survivor values. Attempting to generate high cardiac output and DO_2 is now seen as misplaced in many patients.

- In septic shock, non-survivors fail to increase their VO_2 when DO_2 is increased therapeutically.[16] This probably relates as much if not more to an inability to increase oxygen extraction and/or a maldistribution of flow as to failure to increase global DO_2.

- Thus efforts should be directed towards restoring normal cardiac function and normal organ perfusion, especially in the elderly or in patients with pre-existing cardiac disease.

- Unfortunately there are problems in measuring individual organ perfusion. Splanchnic perfusion is important in septic shock, can be inferred from pHi (see Chapter 1) but is not predictable from global measurements in septic shock.

Inotropic and vasopressor support in septic shock (see also Chapter 8)

- Dobutamine[17] is the inotropic agent of choice for optimizing cardiac output (and therefore global organ blood flow). Excessive rates of infusion may be detrimental.

- Once output is satisfactory, perfusion pressure may be maintained by judicious use of noradrenaline. In septic shock with abnormal vasodilation, the appropriate, i.e. minimal amount, of noradrenaline to maintain SVR and BP without causing excessive vasoconstriction has been shown to increase urine output and promote maintenance of renal function.[18] In severe cases, noradrenaline can reverse refractory septic shock. Noradenaline also improves RV function in septic shock.[19]

- Adrenaline has also been investigated in septic shock and can exert a beneficial effect on haemodynamics[20] – presumably due to its combined inotropic and vasopressors properties. Recent evidence suggests that adrenaline impairs splanchnic perfusion in septic patients compared with noradrenaline and dobutamine and that adding dobutamine infusion to an adrenaline regime improves splanchnic perfusion.[21]

- Dopamine was an early choice for treatment of septic shock in many centres. Dopamine has been shown to be less effective than noradrenaline in restoring haemodynamic parameters and may also reduce splanchnic perfusion compared to noradrenaline.[22]

- The combination of fluid therapy, dobutamine and noradrenaline has much to commend it and is the standard, modern approach in many centres.

Neutralizing the effects of toxins and mediator blockade

- These remain experimental at present.

- It is suggested that haemofiltration may remove toxins and inflammatory mediators from the plasma but at the moment this is controversial.[23]

- An early attempt to block the effect of endotoxin was using the monoclonal antibody to endotoxin, centoxin. Despite initial encouraging results, controlled studies led to the commercial withdrawal of this compound.[24]

- Therefore interest at present is more focused on blocking the cytokine mediated inflammatory cascade. Unfortunately, despite many studies and large financial investment none have fulfilled their theoretical promise. The current state of research is reviewed elsewhere.[25]

Other experimental therapies

- Ibuprofen and other NSAIDs have been investigated for their effects on prostaglandin synthesis but their effects have been disappointing.

- Likewise, although administration of high doses of naloxone result in symptomatic improvement in haemodynamics, long-term improvement and alteration of the course of the disease is unlikely.

- More promising perhaps is work on isolation and production of bactericidal permeability increasing protein which avidly binds to endotoxin and kills bacteria, but this has mainly been used in animal studies so far.

- Arginine analogues are being studied which competitively inhibit the enzyme nitric oxide synthase. There are only case reports and animal studies to date. Controlled trials are eagerly awaited.

- Methylene blue may also inhibit the actions of nitric oxide by inhibiting the target enzyme for nitric oxide action in the endothelium, guanylate cyclase. Haemodynamic parameters can be dramatically improved[26] but the development of pulmonary hypertension may limit the usefulness of this and the arginine analogues.

- Historically corticosteroids have been given in septic shock but two large, controlled, multicentre studies from the USA have failed to demonstrate any beneficial effect. At present the administration of steroids in septic shock is not indicated.[27]

Prognostic indicators

Poor outcome is associated with:

- Increased age.

- Degree of lactic acidaemia, i.e. degree of tissue hypoxia.

- Delay in antibiotic administration, or resistance developing.

- Immunosuppression, e.g. by chemotherapy or, more commonly, corticosteroids.

- Degree of elevation and persistence of cytokine levels.

- Poor prognosis if immunoglobulin levels reduced or low WCC.

- The development of multiple organ failure and the number of organ systems failed.

- The magnitude of the reduction in SVR is claimed by some workers to be the single most important determinant of mortality.[9]

Further Reading

Parrillo JE. Pathogenetic mechanisms of septic shock. *N Engl J Med* 1993; **328**: 1471–7.

Bone RC, Grodzin CJ, Balk RA. Sepsis: a new hypothesis for pathogenesis of the disease process. *Chest* 1997; **112**: 235–43.

Rodeberg DA, Chaet MS, Bass RC *et al*. Nitric oxide: an overview. *Am J Surg* 1995; **170**: 292–303.

Rudis MI, Basha MA, Zarowitz BJ. Is it time to reposition vasopressor and inotropes in sepsis ? *Crit Care Med* 1996; **24**: 525–37.

Zeni F, Freeman B, Natanson C. Anti-inflammatory therapies to treat sepsis and septic shock: a reassessment. *Crit Care Med* 1997; **25**: 1095–100.

References

1. American College of Chest Physicians/Society of Critical Care Medicine Consensus Conference: Definitions for sepsis and organ failure and guidelines for the use of innovative therapies in sepsis. *Crit Care Med* 1992; **20**: 864–74.

2. Rangel-Frausto MS, Pittet D, Costigan M *et al*. The natural history of the systemic inflammatory response syndrome (SIRS). A prospective study. *JAMA* 1995; **273**: 117–23.

3. Muckart DJJ, Bhagwanjee S. American College of Chest Physicians/Society of Critical care Medicine Consensus Conference definitions of the systemic inflammatory response syndrome and allied disorders in relation to critically injured patients. *Crit Care Med* 1997; **25**: 1789–95.

4. Blackwell TS, Christman JW. Sepsis and cytokines: current status. *Br J Anaesth* 1996; **77**: 110–17.

5. Patel RT, Deen KI, Youngs D *et al*. Interleukin 6 is a prognostic indicator of outcome in severe intra-abdominal sepsis. *Br J Surg* 1994; **81**: 1306–8.

6. Parker MM, McCarthy KE, Ognibene FP, Parrillo JE. Right ventricular dysfunction and dilatation, similar to left ventricular changes, characterize the cardiac depression of septic shock in humans. *Chest* 1990; **97**: 126–31.

7. Reilly JM, Cunnion RE, Burch-Whitman C *et al*. A circulating myocardial depressant substance is associated with cardiac dysfunction and peripheral hypoperfusion (lactic acidemia) in patients with septic shock. *Chest* 1989; **95**: 1072–80.

8. Finkel MS, Oddis CV, Jacob TD *et al*. Negative inotropic effects of cytokines on the heart mediated by nitric oxide. *Science* 1992; **257**: 387–9.

9. Groeneveld AB, Nauta JJ, Thijs LG. Peripheral vascular resistance in septic shock: its relation to outcome. *Int Care Med* 1988; **14**: 141–7.

10. Friedman G, Berlot G, Kahn RJ, Vincent JL. Combined measurements of blood lactate concentrations and gastric intramucosal pH in patients with severe sepsis. *Crit Care Med* 1995; **23**: 1184–93.

11. Jardin F, Brun-Ney D, Auvert B *et al*. Sepsis-related cardiogenic shock. *Crit Care Med* 1990; **18**: 1055–60.

12. Reynolds HN, Haupt MT, Thill-Baharozian MC, Carlson RW. Impact of critical care physician staffing on patients with septic shock in a university hospital medical intensive care unit. *JAMA* 1988; **260**: 3446–50.

13. Natanson C, Danner RL, Reilly JM *et al*. Antibiotics versus cardiovascular support in a canine model of human septic shock. *Am J Physiol* 1990; **259**: 1440–7.

14. Schneider AJ, Teule GJ, Groeneveld AB *et al*. Biventricular performance during volume loading in patients with early septic shock, with emphasis on the right ventricle: a combined hemodynamic and radionuclide study. *Am Heart J* 1988; **116**: 103–12.

15. Hayes MA, Timmins AC, Yau EH *et al*. Elevation of systemic oxygen delivery in the treatment of critically ill patients. *N Engl J Med* 1994; **330**: 1717–22.

16. Hayes MA, Timmins AC, Yau EHS. Oxygen transport patterns in patients with sepsis syndrome or septic shock: influence of treatment and relationship to outcome. *Crit Care Med* 1997; **25**: 926–36.

17. Vincent JL, Roman A, Kahn RJ. Dobutamine administration in septic shock: addition to a standard protocol. *Crit Care Med* 1990; **18**: 689–93.

18. Redl-Wenzl EM, Armbruster C, Edelmann G *et al*. The effects of norepinephrine on hemodynamics and renal function in severe septic shock states. *Int Care Med* 1993; **19**: 151–4.

19. Martin C, Perrin G, Saux P *et al*. Effects of norepinephrine on right ventricular function in septic shock patients. *Int Care Med* 1994; **20**: 444–7.

20. Mackenzie SJ, Kapadia F, Nimmo GR *et al*. Adrenaline in treatment of septic shock: effects on haemodynamics and oxygen transport. *Int Care Med* 1991; **17**: 36–9.

21. Levy B, Bollaert PE, Luchelli JP *et al*. Dobutamine improves the adequacy of gastric mucosal perfusion in epinephrine-treated septic shock. *Crit Care Med* 1997; **25**: 1649–54.

22. Marik PE, Mohedin M. The contrasting effects of dopamine and norepinephrine on systemic and splanchnic oxygen utilization in hyperdynamic sepsis. *JAMA* 1994; **272**: 1354–7.

23. Schetz M. Evidence-based analysis of the role of hemofiltration in sepsis and multiorgan dysfunction syndrome. *Curr Opin Crit Care* 1997; **3**: 434–41.

24. McCloskey RV, Straube RC, Sanders C *et al*. Treatment of septic shock with human monoclonal antibody HA-1A. A randomized, double-blind, placebo-controlled trial. CHESS Trial Study Group. *Ann Intern Med* 1994; **121**: 1–5.

25. Zeni F, Freeman B, Natanson C. Anti-inflammatory therapies to treat sepsis and septic shock: a reassessment. *Crit Care Med* 1997; **25**: 1095–100.

26. Gachot B, Bedos JP, Veber B *et al*. Short-term effects of methylene blue on hemodynamics and gas exchange in humans with septic shock. *Int Care Med* 1995; **21**: 1027–31.

27. Lefering R, Neugebauer EA. Steroid controversy in sepsis and septic shock: a meta-analysis. *Crit Care Med* 1995; **23**: 1294–303.

16

ACUTE RENAL FAILURE

R. Kishen

INTRODUCTION

- Acute renal failure (ARF) in the critically ill has high mortality.

- Understanding the applied physiology of the kidney and the pathophysiology of ARF in the critically ill can reduce the incidence of this disease, provide logical guidelines for management of patients at risk of developing ARF as well as improve the outcome.

- It is difficult to estimate the incidence of ARF as the definitions, patient population studied and timing of intervention is different in different studies.

- There is no universally accepted definition of ARF. I suggest a reduction in urine volume to <0.25 ml/kg/h along with a rise in creatinine of >20% and/or the development of metabolic acidosis. The reported incidence varies from 0.14% in 'community acquired' to 33% in ICU settings. Based on 1996/97 (unpublished) data, the incidence of ARF in my ICU was ~25%.

- Lack of sensitive and accurate tests for developing renal dysfunction make the diagnosis difficult in precise terms. Traditional tests include blood biochemistry, urine analysis (unless the patient is anuric) and a high index of suspicion. Recent work[1] on the reintroduction of the 'rate constant' for the clearance of an ideal filterable substance and its measurement non-invasively may allow us to study renal function in real time by the bedside and provide newer insights into ARF.

ARF IN THE CRITICALLY ILL PATIENT (ESPECIALLY THOSE WITH SEPSIS) – A SPECIAL DISEASE?

- ARF in the ICU setting is a 'distinct' disease from that found in the nephrology wards.

- ARF in the critically ill is usually part of multiple organ dysfunction syndrome or MODS[2] and rarely an isolated single organ disease (cf. patients admitted to the nephrology wards – the 'medical' ARF).

- Most cases of ARF are now found in the ICU rather than on general medical wards.[3]

- It is often associated with sepsis, is multifactorial in aetiology (e.g. a combination of sepsis and hypovolaemia) and has a high mortality rate (60–95%).[4]

- Our knowledge of the pathology of ARF in the critically ill is as yet incomplete for many reasons (e.g. due to the lack of biopsy specimens).

- On the other hand the 'medical' ARF usually is a single organ disease, has a low mortality (~8%) and often is the result of a distinct insult (e.g. autoimmune disease, drug toxicity, etc.). Surviving patients recovering from ARF in the ICU usually do not require long-term renal support whereas in 'medical' ARF many patients progress to chronic renal failure.

Applied renal physiology

- Kidneys have a high blood flow (~20–30% of cardiac output, ~400 ml/g tissue) compared with other organs. This high blood flow is primarily for producing glomerular filtrate and is not determined by the kidney's metabolic (oxygen) demand. The renal vasculature is complex and there are regional blood flow variations in the kidney; cortex being well supplied compared with the medulla. The glomerulus is supplied by afferent arteriole; the blood drains by the efferent arteriole, which then supplies the peritubular capillaries (cortical nephrons) or the vasa recta (juxta-glomerular nephrons).

- Under 'normal' conditions renal blood flow (RBF) is autoregulated (i.e. the flow remains constant over a range of blood pressures). The most likely explanation for this is the existence of local myogenic factors regulating RBF. Tubulo-glomerular feedback (TGF) is responsible as well. The mechanisms for autoregulation are still a matter of debate.[5]

- Systemic blood pressure is not a good guide to adequacy of renal blood flow (i.e. perfusion). During hypovolaemia, the kidneys act as the 'blood pressure regulator' (because of renin–angiotensin mechanism) and may be severely hypoperfused despite the blood pressure well within the 'autoregulatory' range.

- The medullary blood flow (especially in the vasa recta) has a low haematocrit (important for the countercurrent mechanism to operate and maintain high osmolality of the medullary interstitium). The low oxygen-carrying capacity of medullary blood, local countercurrent mechanisms (including that for oxygen!) and high osmolality of the medullary interstitium make it a very hostile environment for the structures within it.

- Proximal tubule (pT) and medullary thick ascending loop of Henlé (mTAL) are metabolically very active (sites of active sodium reabsorption) and therefore high consumers of oxygen. Of renal oxygen consumption, 80% is utilized for sodium reabsorption, >90% of which takes place in pT and mTAL. These metabolically demanding structures are in the outer medulla and hence are most vulnerable to hypoxic damage. Medullary hypoxia is the price for efficient urinary concentration by the kidney.

The integrity of the renal excretory function (dependent in most part on RBF) is ensured by a number of local reflex mechanisms:

- afferent and efferent arteriolar smooth muscle – and their control;

- efferent arteriolar constriction to maintain filtration pressure in the glomerulus;

- balance and interplay between dilatory (prostacyclin) and constricting (thromboxane A2) prostanoids;

- interplay between the release of nitric oxide (NO) and endothelin under different conditions;

- TGF.

TGF: an active mechanism for nephron survival

After the loop of Henlé, the tubule passes through the angle between the afferent and efferent arterioles as they enter and emerge from the glomerulus. At this point, specialized tubular cells (macula densa) and the specialized arteriolar smooth muscle cells (granular cells) together form the juxta-glomerular apparatus (jGA).

- With increased glomerular filtrate, jGA is stimulated to release vasoactive substances that cause afferent arteriolar constriction and reduction in the filtrate.

- With low glomerular filtrate, the opposite takes place along with efferent arteriolar constriction (to increase filtration pressure as well).

The nature of these vasoactive substances released is as yet unclear; they are likely to be endothelin, bradykinin, NO and other prostanoids. In situations of low oxygen delivery to the medulla, TGF operates to reduce glomerular filtration. This has two important effects.

- Preservation of fluid because the commonest cause of reduced oxygen delivery to the kidneys is hypoperfusion consequent upon 'hypovolaemia'.

- Reduction of metabolic demand on the proximal nephron (especially mTAL) by reducing the obligatory sodium reabsorption.

Thus the TGF is a mechanism operating to protect the nephron when its metabolic demands cannot be met because of hypoperfusion. This is a very important fact to remember in patients with renal dysfunction.

Mechanisms causing medullary hypoxaemia

Medullary hypoxaemia is the main cause of ARF which is seen clinically as decreased glomerular filtrate (and urine volume). The commonest causes of this are hypovolaemia of any aetiology, low perfusion pressure and sepsis.

- Fluid and blood loss, if not replaced promptly, cause decreased renal blood flow irrespective of blood pressure value.

- Low cardiac output has a similar effect.

- Combined effects of hypovolaemia and low cardiac output (critically low oxygen delivery) have devastating consequences for any organ especially the kidneys.

- Low renal perfusion has a variable effect on different regions of the kidney.

- Although glomerular filtration may be maintained in the early stages, hypovolaemia reduces blood flow in the vasa recta, hence to medulla.

- TGF comes into play to preserve integrity of nephron by reducing its metabolic demand.

Many conditions predispose to medullary hypoxic injury:

- Increased medullary oxygen demand:

  - nephronal hypertrophy in chronic renal disease;

  - solute diuresis as in diabetes, mannitol, hypercalcaemia, radio-contrast agents, dopamine, polyene antibiotics.

- Medullary hypoperfusion:

  - altered structure/compression, e.g. obstructive uropathy, chronic renal failure, atherosclerosis;

  - impaired NO production, e.g. elderly, atherosclerosis, hypertension, pigment nephropathy (myoglobin);

- Impaired prostaglandin synthesis, e.g. non-steroidal anti-inflammatory drugs (NSAID);

- rheological factors, e.g. endotoxin, dehydration, sickle cell anaemia, malaria, radiological contrast media;

- excessive endothelin production, e.g. hypoxia, cyclosporin, endotoxaemia, other cytokines from sepsis, trauma and inflammation.

Endothelin not only initiates ARF but also seems to act to maintain renal dysfunction.

Risk factors that cause increased incidence of ARF, especially after major surgery and/or sepsis

Under normal circumstances 'a single, short insult' does not result in ARF in patients with previously normal renal function. However, repeated and prolonged insults will produce renal dysfunction and if corrective measures are not taken the patient is more likely to develop ARF. A single insult may be enough to produce ARF in the 'population at risk'. Factors that predispose development of ARF are listed as:

- pre-existing renal dysfunction;

- older patients are more prone to develop ARF;

- hypertension, peripheral vascular disease;

- pre-existing cardiac failure (even when cardiac failure is well compensated);

- sepsis especially persistent and unrecognized sepsis;

- diabetes, hypercalcaemia;

- diuretic abuse including frusemide, mannitol and 'renal dose dopamine';

- various antibiotics, e.g. aminoglycosides (gentamicin, etc.), polyenes (e.g. amphotericin);

- X-ray contrast media;

- haem and haem-containing molecules (myoglobin);

- hypovolaemia of any cause (blood, fluid and protein loss).

Prevention of ARF in the critically ill

- Aggressive and proactive management is important in these patients.

- It is better to prevent ARF than to treat it.

- By far the commonest problem causing ARF in the critically ill is inadequate perfusion. For adequate resuscitation (fluids, blood, inotropes) invasive monitoring is usually needed (notwithstanding the controversy about use of pulmonary artery catheters).

- The second commonest cause of ARF in the critically ill is associated sepsis. A thorough search for sepsis in the critically ill is as important as adequate resuscitation. If sepsis is found then the best way to treat it is to drain it if surgically accessible.

- Appropriate antibiotics (with monitoring of toxic antibiotics), nutrition and other supportive therapy complete the picture of strategies for preventing ARF. However, 'prophylactic' antibiotics are often not necessary, are given inadequately and should be limited to one or two large doses. Unnecessary antibiotic use causes more problems than it solves.

- Other causes that contribute to development of ARF in the critically ill are the use of so-called 'renal protective agents' like 'renal dose dopamine' (see below).

- Newer therapies, e.g. calcium channel blockers, adenosine antagonists, prostaglandins, atrial natriuretic factor, etc., have all been tried but have not shown any promise. Endothelin antagonists have so far been encouraging.

Dopamine

Low ('renal') dose dopamine is used in patients with low urine output to augment urine formation. It is also used in 'at risk' patients and after major surgery (e.g. major vascular surgery) to 'reduce' incidence of ARF but there is no convincing evidence that dopamine has or can prevent ARF in these situations.[6]

Dopamine can induce increase in urine production by various mechanisms:

- It can cause increase in cardiac output (especially if hepatic blood flow is reduced, thereby decreasing metabolism of dopamine and therefore its elimination) and thus increase renal blood flow.

- Under the conditions where dopamine may be used, renal vasculature is usually maximally compensating to maintain glomerular filtration rate (GFR) (afferent arteriole is maximally dilated – 'pre-prerenal failure!'). Adding small doses of dopamine will have little, if any, effect.

- Dopamine has a direct effect on the tubular cells to reduce sodium reabsorption – direct diuretic effect. This unabsorbed sodium is presented to the tubule downstream (e.g. mTALs) and thus increases energy expenditure (and therefore oxygen consumption) of that part of the tubule.

Thus dopamine interferes with or abolishes TGF, which can induce tubular damage. The diuretic effect may also worsen hypovolaemia!

- Thus dopamine increases renal blood flow without improving renal tubular oxygen consumption.

- There is no place for unscientific therapies like 'renal dose dopamine' in prevention or management of ARF in the critically ill.

Augmentation of renal perfusion pressure

Volume resuscitation alone may not be sufficient to increase mean arterial pressure in the critically ill. Catecholamines like adrenaline or noradrenaline may have to be used. The use of these drugs may seem illogical especially when noradrenaline infusions are used to produce experimental renal failure. However, renal insults impair renal autoregulation. The renal blood flow then becomes dependent on the perfusion pressure. Experience has shown that with mean arterial pressures >70 mmHg, urine production increases provided the cardiac output can be maintained.

Mannitol

Mannitol is often suggested as a 'renal protective' agent due to its osmotic diuretic, free radical scavenger and renal vasodilatory effect. However:

- in many experimental settings, mannitol has reduced glomerular filtration;

- in most situations reporting beneficial effects of mannitol also involve generous fluid loading!;

- its diuretic effect places unnecessary solute burden on the nephron;

- prospective randomized studies in man have not shown any clear beneficial effect – rather they have underlined the importance of cardiovascular resuscitation and fluid loading.

Frusemide

Frusemide acts on the loop of Henle and reduces chloride, hence sodium reabsorption. This reduces tubular oxygen demand. In situations where there is reduced oxygen supply to the kidney, diuretic therapy with frusemide will produce natriuresis without compromising tubular integrity.

- Frusemide is of theoretical benefit through a reduction in medullary work; prospective randomized studies have not shown any clinical advantage other than yet again point to importance of fluid loading.

- In experimental situations frusemide has shown dramatic decrease in morphological damage.

- Some studies have shown that continuous infusion of frusemide rather than boluses is beneficial as bolus doses may induce further hypovolaemia. Others have failed to demonstrate any difference between the two methods. However:

- large doses of frusemide are 'toxic' to underperfused kidney;

- frusemide can increase the toxicity of certain drugs like aminoglycoside antibiotics;

- studies that have shown beneficial effects of frusemide on the kidney have had large volumes of fluids administered to the patients as part of the protocol;

- there is little evidence that using frusemide (either in boluses or as an infusion) prevents ARF.

There is no benefit of trying to convert 'oliguric' renal failure into 'non-oliguric' renal failure in the critically ill. Often this strategy will not work; moreover there is no difference in mortality rates in the two forms of ARF despite increased urine output in non-oliguric renal failure.

Management of ARF

Management of ARF in the critically ill is not restricted to the kidneys; the whole patient management of MODS is the only way to treat these patients. Therefore, therapeutic strategies suitable for MODS are equally well suited for ARF along with the addition of renal supportive therapy.

Resuscitation

- Hypoperfusion must be considered in all critically ill patients.

- Hypoperfusion may be obvious – low blood pressure, low cardiac output but evaluation of perfusion may be difficult and other parameters may have to be considered, e.g. base excess, lactate, gastric intramucosal pH, oxygen delivery and consumption. The adequacy of resuscitation/perfusion should be assessed frequently and changes made in therapy as necessary.

- Fluids, blood and inotropes – used appropriately may all be necessary.

- Invasive cardiovascular monitoring will be of advantage but is not absolutely essential (depends upon the patient's condition).

Treatment of sepsis

- Infections may be obvious or occult.

- Appropriate antibiotics must be given; may often have to be given empirically after culture samples of various body fluids (including blood) have been taken.

- Antibiotic therapy must be reviewed in light of the microbiological investigations' results and the advice of microbiologists is invaluable.

- Treat surgically accessible sepsis by appropriate operation but operations are only performed after resuscitation and cardiovascular stabilization. The patient may need further resuscitation and/or stabilization after the operation.

Surveillance for and detection of further infection or perfusion deficit must continue as part of overall supportive therapy. Other aspects of supportive therapy are important, e.g. nutrition, as discussed elsewhere.

Renal supportive therapy

Here any form of supportive therapy for renal dysfunction will be referred to as renal replacement therapy (RRT) and any continuous form of RRT will be referred to as CRRT. For the critically ill, continuous rather than intermittent forms of RRT are better tolerated and clinically beneficial.

- Once the ARF is established or imminent little is gained by delaying the RRT.

- The actual form of RRT will depend upon:

  - the patient's condition;

  - the equipment available;

  - the skill and experience of the medical and nursing staff in attendance.

- On no account should RRT or CRRT be undertaken without proper understanding of the equipment and proper skills by those using the equipment, otherwise great harm can result to the patients.

- Available methods for RRT are:

  - intermittent haemodialysis (as that for chronic renal failure patients) with or without ultrafiltration;

  - slow continuous ultrafiltration (SCUF);

  - arteriovenous haemofiltration (CAVH – also called 'spontaneous' or 'non-pumped' haemofiltration);

  - venovenous haemofiltration (CVVH – also called 'pumped' haemofiltration);

- arterio- or venovenous haemodiafiltration (CAVHD or CVVHD; occasionally to avoid confusion with continuous forms of dialysis it is also called CAVHDF or CVVHDF).

It is important to understand the physical principles involved in different forms of RRT to get the maximum clinical benefit. Diffusion of solute down a concentration gradient is the basic working principle in dialysis (intermittent or continuous forms). This requires a relatively high blood flow on one side and a dialysate flow on the other side of a semipermeable membrane. Haemofiltration on the other hand works on the principle of 'convective' transfer where the plasma water (without its protein) and the water-soluble solute pass through a semipermeable membrane as the 'ultrafiltrate'.

The haemofilter, thus, resembles a collection of glomeruli (where filtration occurs) but without the accompanying tubules (where the reabsorption can occur).

- In dialysis, the creatinine clearance mainly depends upon the blood flow through the dialyser.

- In haemofiltration, the creatinine clearance depends upon the amount of the ultrafiltrate produced.[7]

It is erroneously assumed that haemofiltration cannot adequately control uraemia (and creatinine levels) in the critically ill because the creatinine clearance of the CVVH system is poorer than CVVHD (or CAVHD). CVVH but not CAVH is an adequate form of CRRT (perhaps even better than CVVHD) in all patients with ARF.[7]

Advantages of CRRT in critically ill patients with ARF

- CRRT is slow and 'gentle' on the cardiovascular system of these unstable patients.

- It allows adequate uraemic control, which is achieved slowly, thus avoiding disequilibration syndrome.

- It allows removal of large quantities of fluid to create a 'space' for the obligatory input of fluid in form of sedation, antibiotics, inotropes and i.v. feed.

- As fluid can be removed slowly and over a long period, physiological 'instability' is avoided.

- Adequate uraemic control is achieved even in very severely catabolic patients.

- The haemofilter membranes (polyacrylonitrile-PAN, polysulphone) are more biocompatible than dialysis membranes.

- There is much less of the patient's blood in the extracorporeal circuit.

- The techniques of CRRT are easy to learn.

- CRRT may have other advantages like removal of cytokines and proinflammatory materials (the 'middle molecules') from the circulation of the critically ill.[8] This is because of the bigger pore size of the filter membrane.

Further reading

Lins RL, Chew SL, Daelemans R. Epidemiology of acute renal failure. In Bellomo R, Ronco C (eds), *Acute Renal Failure in the Critically Ill*. Berlin: Springer, 1995, pp. 147–59.

Lote CJ, Harper L, Savage COS. Mechanisms of acute renal failure. *Br J Anaesth* 1996; **77**: 82–9.

Bersten AD, Holt AW. Prevention of acute renal failure in the critically ill patient. In Bellomo R, Ronco C (eds), *Acute Renal Failure in the Critically Ill*. Berlin: Springer, 1995, pp. 122–46.

References

1. Rabito CA, Moore RH, Bougas C, Dragotakes SC. Noninvasive, real time monitoring of the renal function: the ambulatory renal monitor. *J Nucl Med* 1993; **34**: 199–207.

2. Elasy TA, Anderson RJ. Changing demography of acute renal failure. *Semin Dial* 1996; **9**: 438–43.

3. Bellomo R, Ronco C. The changing pattern of severe acute renal failure. *Nephrology* 1996; **2**: 149–54.

4. Ronco C, Bellomo R. The rising era of critical care nephrology. *Curr Opin Crit Care* 1997; **3**: 405–7.

5. Steinhausen M, Endlich K, Wiegman DL. Glomerular blood flow. *Kidney International* 1990; **38**: 769–84.

6. Cottee DB, Saul WP. Is renal dose dopamine protective or therapeutic? No. *Crit Care Clin* 1996; **12**: 687–95.

7. Brocklehurst IC, Thomas AN, Kishen R, Guy JM. Creatinine and urea clearance during continuous veno-venous haemofiltration in critically ill patients. *Anaesthesia* 1996; **51**: 551–3.

8. Schetz M. Evidence-based analysis of the role of hemofiltration in sepsis and multiorgan dysfunction syndrome. *Curr Opin Crit Care* 1997: **3**: 434–41.

17

ACUTE RESPIRATORY DISTRESS SYNDROME

C. Clarke

DEFINITION

The definition of ARDS remains controversial. This has led to dispute as to the incidence and outcome of the syndrome.

- A current, widely held view is that the term ARDS should be reserved for those patients at the severe end of an 'Acute Lung Injury (ALI)' spectrum. (ARDS had previously been widely known as *Adult* Respiratory distress syndrome.)

- An alternate view is that ARDS patients have ALI and also have increased pulmonary vascular permeability or 'Diffuse Alveolar Damage'.[1] Measurements of permeability, however, are not routine.

DIAGNOSIS

- Various groups have proposed criteria for the diagnosis of ARDS, usually these include:[2]

- the presence of a recognized risk factor;

- an index of the degree of hypoxia (PaO_2/FiO_2, shunt fraction);

- the presence of pulmonary infiltrates; and

- the exclusion of cardiogenic pulmonary oedema (often by specifying an arbitrary maximum pulmonary artery wedge pressure).

- The Murray Lung Injury Score[3] (LIS) is widely used in the literature, having four components (not all of which need be assessed). A score is assigned for:

  - hypoxia;

- lung infiltrates;
- level of PEEP;
- pulmonary compliance.

The total score is then divided by the number of components measured to give the LIS. A LIS >2.5 is accepted as denoting severe ALI or ARDS.

- In reading the literature the term 'ECMO entry criteria' is often encountered. This refers to the National Institutes of Health (NIH) extracorporeal oxygenation study of 1974–77. Patients fulfilling ECMO criteria have an extremely high mortality. the criteria are:

  - fast entry PaO_2 <50 mmHg at $FiO_2 = 1.0$;
  - PEEP >5 cmH_2O;
  - slow entry PaO_2 <50 mmHg at $FiO_2 = 0.6$;
  - PEEP >5 cmH_2O;
  - plus shunt fraction >30% ($FiO_2 = 1.0$), all after 48 h on ICU.

- Precise definitions of ARDS may become more important as new potential therapies are targeted against ARDS or its predispositions.

PREDISPOSITIONS TO ARDS

In the early 1980s several groups looked at risk factors for ARDS.[4] In fact if we regard ARDS as 'shock lung', intuitively almost any cause of shock or of neutrophil activation is capable of triggering the syndrome. Some predispositions have declined in importance – oxygenator technology now means that uncomplicated cardiopulmonary bypass is an unusual cause of ARDS. Several important lessons remain:

- Sepsis is probably the commonest predisposition.
- Multiple predispositions confer dramatically increased risk (underlined by the 85% risk of developing ARDS in the setting of the septic burns patient who requires a massive transfusion).
- Outcome is dramatically influenced by the underlying predisposition. This was dramatically illustrated in the European ARDS study – many ARDS patients die of their underlying disease or its complications.[5]
- In general ARDS following aspiration or trauma will have a better prognosis than ARDS complicating sepsis.

Incidence

Estimates of ARDS incidence vary considerably (due in part to differing definitions). The NHLI study from the USA put the incidence at 60/100,000 – surprisingly high figure. More recent estimates from the Canary Islands, Spain (in an attempt to identify a discrete population) and from Yorkshire were between 1.5 and 4.5/100,000.[6,7] ARDS forms a major part of the workload in a typical ICU – ~14% of ventilated patients will have a LIS >2.5.

Aetiology

Three phases of ARDS are described:

- Initial injury.
- Exudative phase.
- Fibroproliferative phase.

The sequence of events is not fully understood. However, there is an early rise in interleukin 8 (IL-8) which can be used as a marker for high risk patients progressing to ARDS.

- Injury can be a direct alveolar injury or can be endothelial mediated as a consequence of a systemic inflammatory reaction. Often there is crossover with an inflammatory aspect of direct injury.

- There is rapid sequestration and activation of leukocytes in the lung – a process involving both circulating neutrophils and alveolar macrophages. Other cytokines – notably IL-1, IL-6 and tumour necrosis factor (TNF) – are also important and can be found at bronchoalveolar lavage (BAL). Persistently elevated concentrations of these cytokines in BAL fluid are associated with poor outcome. There is evidence that ventilatory management might alter the cytokine release pattern.

- Once sequestered leukocytes can release toxic products such as oxygen radicals and proteases. Lung damage and gap formation in the alveolar-capillary membrane follow. The natural defence systems – superoxide dismutase, catalase and glutathione peroxidase – are lacking in the ARDS lung.

- Myofibroblasts can migrate through the gaps and lay down connective tissue on the alveolar side of the basement membrane. Subsequent remodelling (or its failure) is important in the development of progressive fibroproliferation. Extracellular matrix components such as collagen and fibronectin are damaged. The possible role of steroids in preventing fibroproliferation is discussed below.

Clinical features

- Mild forms of ALI can sometimes be managed with CPAP by a face mask. Patients with ARDS nearly always require IPPV.

- There may be an initial latent period but respiratory distress develops within 12–72 h of the predisposing event.

- There is severe hypoxia, unrelieved by oxygen therapy, increased work of breathing and reduced pulmonary compliance.

- The degree of hypoxia may seem out of proportion to the radiological features in the early stages but later CXRs may show widespread bilateral infiltrates – the classic 'whiteout'.

- Late stages of ARDS are often characterized by pulmonary hypertension and right ventricle (RV) dysfunction.[8]

Management

- Management of ARDS is essentially supportive and should involve treatment of the underlying condition along with a ventilatory strategy that minimizes further lung injury.

- Infection, ventilator-induced lung injury (barotrauma and volutrauma) and fibroproliferation are common complications and can be difficult to diagnose.

- Infection can be clinically indistinguishable from fibroproliferation, hence interest in techniques such as protected brochoalveolar lavage and protected brushing.

- The chest X-ray may fail to identify significant pneumothoraces and surveillance CT scanning may be necessary.

- Before describing recent advances that are not *proven* to alter ARDS mortality it is important to emphasize the importance of meticulous basic ICU management in this condition.

Ventilatory strategy (see also Chapters 6 and 7)

- Pressure volume loops demonstrate a characteristic inflection point in early ARDS. Above this 'lower inflection point' the lung compliance increases. Traditional methods of ventilating on the most compliant part of the curve involve either the use of large tidal volumes or the titration of PEEP to abolish the lower inflection point – one of the so-called 'best PEEP' techniques.

- The concept of an 'ideal' level of PEEP is simplistic – the PEEP required to keep open a lung region equals the hydrostatic forces acting over (compressing) that region, these forces increase towards dependent lung regions which therefore have a different 'ideal' PEEP. One may need to combine PEEP titration with tidal volume reduction as non-dependent lung regions may be close to their 'upper inflection point' (a flattening of the P/V curve signalling over distension) even at the start of inspiration.

- Reversed I:E ratio ventilation is commonly utilized and frequently results in auto- or intrinsic PEEP which allows alveolar recruitment. A prolonged inspiration may allow recruitment of alveoli with long time constants. As auto-PEEP is only applied to lung units participating in ventilation, the dead space/tidal volume ratio falls. The utilization of auto-PEEP may be less damaging than applied PEEP and many authorities consider pressure-controlled reverse ratio ventilation (PCIRV) as the optimum way to ventilate in acute lung injury.

- PEEP, both auto- and applied, may protect lung units from shear injury caused by repetitive collapse and reopening – so called 'low end barotrauma'. In terms of alveolar recruitment, our ventilatory aims are thus to 'open up the lung and keep it open'.

- Gattinoni and Pelosi[9] combined measurements of respiratory mechanics with CT images and advanced the concept of the 'baby lung'. On CT some lung areas are densely consolidated, while others appear normal. Three zones can be described – closed diseased, open diseased and recruitable. The total open plus recruitable volume is small – a 'baby' lung – and is vulnerable to damage from an excess tidal volume as its specific compliance is relatively normal. Consolidated lung predominates in dependent zones, but can redistribute.

- From this concept various volume and pressure-limiting strategies have evolved. These include:

  - ventilation with small tidal volumes and permissive hypercapnia;

  - pressure-controlled ventilation;

  - the encouragement of spontaneous modes;

  - extracorporeal carbon dioxide removal (and intravascular oxygenation).

- Enthusiasm for permissive hypercapnia was high, and mortality is reported to be lower than expected.[10] Hypercapnia can be problematic. Permissive hypercapnia is contraindicated in the head-injured patient and possibly in patients with ischaemic heart disease. Pulmonary hypertension is exacerbated. Nevertheless, many clinicians now consider pressures and volumes to be more important than achieving 'normal' levels of carbon dioxide.

Adjunctive therapy

Adjunctive therapies may help correct V/Q mismatch without further ventilator-induced lung injury. Some have long been abandoned, e.g. early high dose steroids, intravenous prostaglandin, ibuprofen. Combinations of adjunctive therapies, e.g. nitric oxide and partial liquid ventilation,[11] may be more beneficial than either alone.

Fluid restriction – 'keeping the lung dry'

Although the rationale may be unduly simplistic, the balance of opinion is probably shifting towards keeping the injured lung dry[12] – with the important proviso that cardiac function and organ perfusion must be maintained. Certainly administration of excessive fluid will be detrimental.

Prone positioning

It is suggested that paralysed patients turned prone will have better expansion of dorsal lung regions with high perfusion, and hence better oxygenation. Subsequent reports in ARDS patients have demonstrated significant improvements in oxygenation allowing reduction of FiO_2 and PEEP, and persisting over days. Unfortunately this improvement is not seen in all patients. The mechanism is difficult to elicit,[13] but

- the prone position may increase FRC;

- hydrostatic forces are important – in Gattinoni's CT studies the closed areas are in dependent lung areas, but rapidly redistribute (30 min) upon turning the patient prone. As oedema is uniformly distributed throughout the lung and the redistribution on turning prone is so rapid the likely explanation is that the heavy oedematous lung is collapsing under its own weight;

- the now non-dependent, better ventilated dorsal regions may also be well perfused as West's gravitational zones may not hold.

Enthusiasm for the prone position with its logistic problems (pressure sores, tube and line displacement, decompensation on being returned to the supine position) varies, in some units prone positioning is routine, in others it is unheard of.

Surfactant in ARDS

- Pulmonary surfactant reduces alveolar surface tension by the formation of a phospholipid monolayer.

- Surfactant is a 90% lipid/10% protein mixture.

- The two functionally most important phospholipids are reduced in ARDS, the reduction correlating with severity.

Early in the development of ARDS plasma proteins leak into the alveolar space and alter the monolayer. Furthermore, as the syndrome progresses surfactant may become incorporated into hyaline membranes. While these changes are reversible a process of 'collapse induration' may occur whereby atelectasis consequent to the surfactant depletion allows approximation of the alveolar walls. Subsequent fibroblast activation may convert the approximated walls to the honeycomb lung characteristic of late fibroproliferative ARDS. This change is irreversible.

Surfactant depletion in the early stages also favours lung oedema formation by decreasing interstitial pressures and therefore decreasing oedema reabsorbtion. Recently there has been increasing appreciation of the decrease in host defences caused by loss of surfactant-associated proteins.

The early changes may be reversible by the administration of exogenous surfactant.

- Exogenous surfactant is either natural (porcine or bovine) or synthetic. It can be administered by direct instillation – the standard method in neonates, or by aerosolization.

- Theoretically the greatest advantage of exogenous surfactant administration would be in early ALI – unfortunately we have no method of determining which patients with lung injury will progress to ARDS. Surfactant administration in the presence of collapse induration may still have a role but cannot reverse the existing damage and it is likely that higher doses (probably by instillation) may be required.

- A multicentre trial using aerosolized surfactant was abandoned due to lack of effect.[14] Both the dose and method of administration have been questioned and a subsequent smaller study using instillation showed benefit.[15]

Partial liquid ventilation (PLV)

Perfluorocarbons (fluorine substituted hydrocarbons) are volatile, have a low surface tension and can carry both O_2 and CO_2. In PLV a dose of perfluorocarbons approximating to the FRC is instilled directly into the lungs and ventilation is carried out using a conventional ventilator. The clinical signs of an adequate dosage are:[16]

- acceptable peak inspiratory pressure; and

- the presence of a meniscus in the ETT (evaporation of perfluorocarbon over time may limit efficacy)

Relatively small doses give maximum surface tension reduction, larger doses redistribute in an inhomogenous manner – preferentially into collapsed, dependent lung areas – leading to alveolar recruitment and enhancing V/Q matching.

Interestingly PLV may decrease lung inflammation, but without a direct effect on neutrophil function. It may be that liquid ventilation reduces barotrauma by decreasing shear stress and preventing end-expiratory collapse. There may also be a lavage effect – this has its cons, as there is relative surfactant deficiency or alteration on weaning from PLV.

Inhaled nitric oxide

- There is a history of administering vasodilators to ARDS patients – pulmonary hypertension being a hallmark of the syndrome.

- Systematically administered vasodilators have failed to be effective, actually increasing Qs/Qt and causing hypotension.

In 1987 two groups working independently showed that 'endothelium-derived relaxing factor' was in fact nitric oxide (NO). We are now aware that NO has a range of biological actions which range from control of vascular tone through neutrophil function and to neurotransmission.

NO is present in air at about 9 ppm, is an environmental pollutant and an important constituent of cigarette smoke. It is highly lipid soluble and rapidly crosses endothelium. In the presence of oxygen NO is oxidized to the highly toxic nitrogen dioxide (NO_2). NO causes the conversion of arginine to citrulline with an increase in intracellular cGMP. This is the case whether it is produced in the body (by a nitric oxide synthase) or inhaled (INO) diffusing through pulmonary endothelial cells. It is rapidly inactivated $(t_{1/2} = 111\text{–}30$ ms) by binding to haemoglobin (producing methaemoglobin and nitrate ion). Numerous observational clinical studies have demonstrated that INO decreases pulmonary artery pressure and shunt.

INO is a selective pulmonary vasodilator being distributed preferentially to lung areas that are ventilated and dilating the pulmonary vasculature in these areas. Theoretically the pulmonary vasculature around true shunt areas is not dilated. The fall in pulmonary artery pressure has further effects:

- There is a fall in oedema formation (reduced hydrostatic pressure).

- Hypoxic pulmonary vasoconstriction (HPV) may become more effective as the pulmonary artery pressure falls.

- Improvement in RV dysfunction[17] commonly associated with ARDS.

PaO_2 improves at a much lower dose than that giving maximum pulmonary artery vasodilatation. Indeed a clinical effect can be seen at 1 ppm.

INO has many limitations:

- Not all patients are responders.

- Delivery is not straightforward.[18]

- There is a toxicity potential both for patients and staff mainly related to nitrogen dioxide (NO_2) production.

- INO cannot be effective in the presence of massive oedema and fibro-proliferation.

- Effects on oxygenation can be demonstrated – effect on outcome is uncertain.

- At higher doses NO may diffuse to consolidated areas and offset the regional HPV (loss of selectivity). Furthermore, NO may bind to albumin and be released downstream causing systemic vasodilation.

- Discontinuation of INO can cause a rebound phenomenon and weaning may be difficult – possibly because endogenous production has been switched off.

The balance of the NO effect and effects of ventilation is important and it is now realised that as much lung recruitment as possible must be achieved in conjunction with INO. Otherwise there is a danger that we could be given a false sense of achievement by the improvement in oxygenation and reduce lung recruiting manoeuvres – with overall detrimental effects in the longer term.

Technically the limitations of continuous delivery systems dictate that they should not be used in the adult. Premixing or inspiratory injection systems are more satisfactory, although premixing allows more time for NO_2 formation and some inspiratory injection systems cope poorly if the flow is not constant (PCV or spontaneous breaths).[19]

Two recent multicentre trials have failed to demonstrate an decrease in mortality in the INO group, and indeed in the European AGA trial initiation of haemofiltration was more frequent in the INO group. A recent American phase II trial found no difference in the frequency of adverse events between placebo and INO groups. In this randomized, double-blinded trial several INO doses were used. Although no difference in mortality was demonstrated (at any dose) the 5 ppm INO patients had a significant improvement in a *post-hoc* analysis of the variable 'alive and off ventilation at 28 days'. This multicentre trial also demonstrated that INO was well tolerated at up to 40 ppm, although selective vasodilation is lost >20 ppm.[20]

Steroids

- Progressive pulmonary fibroproliferation (PFP) is probably, directly or indirectly, the major cause of death in ARDS. PFP not only causes hypoxic death but also by increasing ventilator days it allows further episodes of ventilator-associated pneumonia (VAP) leading to sepsis and organ failure. Fibroproliferation is the only cause of fever in 25% of ARDS patients.

- Preventing PFP is obviously attractive and attempts have been made using sustained courses of steroids. PFP is variously diagnosed by the presence of fever, increased uptake on gallium citrate scanning and on open lung biopsy. The major differential diagnosis is VAP and surveillance bronchial brushing or protected lavage may have a role.

- Meduri *et al.*[21] found three patterns of response to sustained steroids – rapid, delayed and non-response. Survival was 86% in responders and only 25% in non-responders. VAP developed more often in non-responders.

- In the past major studies have underlined the potential for septic complications when ARDS patients are given steroids and these promising results must be treated with caution.

Extracorporeal life support

Extracorporeal life support (ELS) aims to support adequate gas exchange while preventing ventilator-induced lung injury.

Extracorporeal membrane oxygenation (ECMO) is similar to cardiopulmonary bypass and usually implies arterial drainage cannulae with venous return. It is highly invasive. The NIH ECMO study (1974–77) in the USA demonstrated an unexpectedly high mortality rate in both the ECMO and the conventional management groups (predicted mortality rate of 65%, observed 91%) and in effect resulted in a moratorium on ECMO in the USA. It did demonstrate that ECMO was effective and that the average survival in ECMO patients was longer than controls.

- Extracorporeal carbon dioxide removal (ECCO$_2$-R) is a modification designed primarily to remove CO$_2$. Thus a high gas flow is used (sometimes with two oxygenators in series), but importantly blood flow can be lower and venovenous cannulation is possible. Although less invasive, full heparinization is still usually necessary and bleeding remains a major complication. Recent advances include percutaneous cannulation and the use of heparin-bonded membranes that help to reduce the transfusion requirement. The Milan experience with ECCO$_2$-R is that mortality is ~50%.

- The intravascular oxygenator (IVOX) places the membrane oxygenator in the vena cava. The current generation of devices cannot decrease the ventilatory requirement, but the technique has great potential. The IVOX device is not currently available but several alternatives such as the pumping artificial lung (PAL) are under development.

All studies, including the most recent randomized controlled study, again have shown extracorporeal techniques to be no better[22] (but no worse) than maximum conventional management. The three major studies do have limitations and safe conclusions are:

- extracorporeal techniques are effective;

- the risk of the technique precludes its use in less ill patients;

- it is essential that expertise is concentrated in a limited number of centres; and

- controversially it has been recommended that ELS is only used in the setting of randomized trials.

Outcome of ARDS

- The majority of deaths are due to sepsis and extrapulmonary organ failures. Outcome worsens with increasing organ failures.

- Classic teaching is that only ~16% of ARDS deaths are due to hypoxia.[23] However, more recent studies have shown progressive respiratory failure to be an important cause of death. One explanation may be that pneumonia has been a common predisposition in those series with a high incidence of progressive respiratory failure. Conceivably pneumonia might sensitize the lung making fibroproliferation and unremitting respiratory failure more likely.

- The NHLI ECMO study conducted from 1974 to 1977 showed the outcome of the control group to be no different from the ECMO group, and the mortality rate to be ~90%. As management became more sophisticated the mortality rate fell to ~70% and remained consistently at this level. Disappointment with lack of progress led to a feeling that the requirement for a rigorous definition ('PARDS', or publishable ARDS) to report a series was selecting out a subset of severely ill patients with a high mortality.

- During the 1990s, reported mortality has been lower, ~50%, and in some isolated series much lower still. Most clinicians are of the opinion that mortality has decreased over the past decade. However, a recent critical examination of all major series with mortality reported does not back up this impression.[24] One explanation would be an increase in age and comorbidity of the general ICU population.

- Most survivors return to reasonably normal lung function though some dysfunction may be detectable by formal pulmonary function testing.[25]

Further reading

Artigas A, Bernard GR, Carlet J et al. The American–European Consensus Conference on ARDS, Part 2. Ventilatory, pharmacologic, supportive therapy, study design strategies and issues related to recovery and remodelling. *Int Care Med* 1998; **24**: 378–98.

Downey GP, Granton JT. Mechanisms of acute lung injury. *Curr Opin Crit Care* 1997; **3**: 43–50.

Lessard MR. New concepts in mechanical ventilation for ARDS. *Can J Anesth* 1996; **43**: R42–54.

Kollef MH, Schuster DP. The acute respiratory distress syndrome. *N Engl J Med* 1995; **332**: 27–37.

References

1. Schuster DP. Identifying patients with ARDS: time for a different approach. *Int Care Med* 1997; **23**: 1197–203.

2. Bernard GR, Artigas A, Brigham KL et al. The American–European Consensus Conference on ARDS: definitions, mechanisms, relevant outcomes, and clinical trial co-ordination. *Am J Respir Crit Care Med* 1994; **149**: 818–24.

3. Murray JF, Mathay MA, Luce JM et al. An expanded definition of the adult respiratory distress syndrome. *Am Rev Respir Dis* 1988; **138**: 720–3.

4. Pepe P, Potkin R, Reus D et al. Clinical predictors of the adult respiratory distress syndrome. *Am J Surg* 1982; **144**: 124–30.

5. Hudson LD, Steinberg KP. Epidemiology of ARDS. Incidence and outcome: a changing picture. In Marini JJ, Evans TW (eds), *Update in Intensive Care and Emergency Medicine*, 30. *Acute Lung Injury*. Berlin: Springer, 1998.

6. Webster NR, Cohen AT, Nunn JF. Adult respiratory distress syndrome – how many cases in the UK? *Anaesthesia* 1988; **43**: 923–6

7. Villar J, Slutsky AS. The incidence of the adult respiratory distress syndrome. *Am Rev Resp Dis* 1989; **140**: 814–16

8. Vincent JL. Is ARDS usually associated with right ventricular dysfunction or failure? *Int Care Med* 1995; **21**: 195–6.

9. Gattinoni L, Pelosi P. Pathophysiologic insights into acute respiratory failure. *Curr Opin Crit Care* 1996; **2**: 8–12

10. Hickling KG, Walsh J, Henderson S *et al*. Low mortality rate in adult respiratory distress syndrome using low-volume, pressure-limited ventilation with permissive hypercapnia: a prospective study. *Crit Care Med* 1994; **22**: 1568–78.

11. Houmes RJ, Hartog A, Verbrugge SJ *et al*. Combining partial liquid ventilation with nitric oxide to improve gas exchange in acute lung injury *Int Care Med* 1997; **23**: 163–9.

12. Schuller D, Schuster DP. Fluid management in acute respiratory distress syndrome. *Curr Opin Crit Care* 1996; **2**: 1–7.

13. Villar J. Adjunctive therapies for the treatment of acute respiratory distress syndrome. *Curr Opin Crit Care* 1998; **4**: 27–35

14. Anzueto A, Baughman RP, Guntupalli KK *et al*. Aerosolized surfactant in adults with sepsis-induced acute respiratory distress syndrome. *N Engl J Med* 1996; **334**: 1417–21.

15. Walmrath D, Gunther A, Ghofrani AG *et al*. Bronchoscopic surfactant administration in patients with severe adult respiratory distress syndrome and sepsis. *Am J Respir Crit Care Med* 1996; **154**: 57–62.

16. Lachman B, Verbrugge S. Liquid ventilation. *Curr Opin Crit Care* 1996; **2**: 60–6.

17. Rossaint R, Slama K, Steudel W *et al*. Effects of inhaled nitric oxide on right ventricular function in severe acute respiratory distress syndrome. *Int Care Med* 1995; **21**: 197–203.

18. Young JD, Dyar OJ. Delivery and monitoring of inhaled nitric oxide. *Int Care Med* 1996; **22**: 77–86.

19. Cuthbertson BH, Dellinger P, Dyar OJ *et al*. UK Guidelines for the use of inhaled nitric oxide therapy in adult ICUs. *Int Care Med* 1997; **23**: 1212–18.

20. Dellinger RP, Zimmerman JL, Taylor RW *et al*. Effects of inhaled nitric oxide in patients with acute respiratory distress syndrome: results of a randomized phase II trial. *Crit Care Med* 1998; **26**: 15–23.

21. Meduri GU, Chinn AJ, Leeper KV. Corticosteroid rescue treatment of progressive fibroproliferation in late ARDS: patterns of response and predictors of outcome. *Chest* 1994; **105**: 1516–27.

22. Morris AH, Wallace CJ, Menlove RL *et al*. Randomised clinical trial of pressure controlled inverse ratio ventilation and extracorporeal CO_2 removal for

adult respiratory distress syndrome. *Am J Respir Crit Care Med* 1994; **149**: 295–300.

23. Montgomery A, Stager M, Carrico C *et al*. Causes of mortality in the adult respiratory distress syndrome. *Am Rev Resp Dis* 1985; **132**: 485–9.

24. Krafft P, Fridrich P, Pernerstorfer T *et al*. The acute respiratory distress syndrome: definitions, severity and clinical outcome. An analysis of 101 clinical investigations. *Int Care Med* 1996; **22**: 519–25.

25. Hudson LD. What happens to survivors of the adult respiratory distress syndrome? *Chest* 1994: **105**: 123S–126S.

18

THE PATIENT WITH GASTROINTESTINAL PROBLEMS

THE GUT AS THE SOURCE OR VICTIM OF MULTIPLE ORGAN FAILURE

Many have suggested that the gut is the source or 'motor' of multiple organ failure. The rationale includes:

- Increased permeability of the gut wall in shock and critical illness. Remember the gut lumen is effectively 'outside' the body. The skin has many layers of protection. The gut lining is much thinner and more vulnerable.

- This permits translocation of bacteria and/or endotoxin into the circulation. Animal studies have clearly shown this to occur. Patient studies are not so convincing with few studies demonstrating translocation as a clinically relevant problem[1] in all but the most extreme, preterminal situations.

- The liver normally (impaired in severe liver dysfunction and severe multiple organ failure) clears these substances from the portal circulation – most of the reticuloendothelial system is in the abdomen. However, this leads to an inflammatory response and cytokine production that, obviously, has systemic effects.

- The gut may be especially sensitive to reperfusion injury (oxygen-free radicals produced when the blood flow to ischaemic tissue is restored). There is certainly an abundance of xanthine dehydrogenase in the gut wall (which is needed for bacterial phagocytosis as part of the gut's defences) that leads to production of the superoxide radical.

- However, the opposing view would suggest that the gut is an 'innocent bystander' in shock every bit as much as the kidney. Gut hypoperfusion or failure may simply *mirror* the development of organ failure rather than precede or cause it. Is the gut merely an early victim in the critically ill patient; is the increased permeability just part of the generalized increases in membrane permeability in critical illness and are gut ischaemia and translocation simply markers of organ failure of the gut which happens to be particularly sensitive?

Therapeutic implications

- Maintaining gut perfusion. pHi may be an indicator of stomach and bowel perfusion adequacy. A low pHi may be restored by fluids,[2] or dobutamine.[3] However, an editorial in *Critical Care Medicine* tried to put pHi and gut ischaemia into perspective. There is a 'considerable jump from suggesting that gut ischaemia may be a good predictor of outcome and that pHi is a true reflection of gut ischaemia and that it may be manipulated – all with scientific work to support them, to implying that gut ischaemia/translocation are a cause of multiple organ failure'.[4]

- Maintain hepatic function (see below).

- Early enteral nutrition. Possible benefit of glutamine for the small bowel and fibre for the large bowel (see Chapter 5).

- Antioxidant and other therapies to protect against reperfusion injury are being evaluated.

Selective digestive decontamination (SDD)

- First reported in 1984.

- The assumption is that major nosocomial pathogens in selected, vulnerable hosts originate in the gastrointestinal (GI) tract and that sterilization of these enteric organisms will reduce nosocomial infection rates and improve outcome in critically ill patients.

- Most published regimens include a cocktail of oral (non-absorbable) antibiotics with a short course of a systemic antibiotic, e.g. a cephalosporin. Confusion has arisen and it has been difficult to compare studies due to differences in reported regimens, e.g. different antibiotic combinations.

- There are enthusiasts who publish regularly but many ICUs remain unconvinced.

- Acceptance has been limited by high costs, labour-intensive regimen, a need for close microbiological support as well as by doubts about efficacy. There are in addition major causes for concern regarding development of long-term antibiotic resistance.

- A limitation is that it can only clear susceptible organisms, with an increase in non-susceptible staphylococci and enterococci in some studies.

- Most studies have shown reductions in nosocomial infections but, in general, overall mortality rates have not been significantly improved apart from highly selected groups of patients, e.g. trauma patients. Meta analyses[5,6] have not been sufficiently convincing to persuade ICUs to undertake this controversial therapy in heterogenous groups of patients.

The problem of resistance

The development of antibiotic resistance has always been a potential problem with SDD. Some studies have failed to find any significant effects but there *are* reports of problem infections from unusual organisms.[7] The potential long-term problems are even more worrying.[8]

- Antibiotic resistance may require prolonged periods before consequences observed, e.g. penicillin-resistant streptococcal pneumonia did not become a clinical problem until nearly 4 decades of β-lactamase use. In past few years, enteroccoci, methicillin-resistant *Staphylococcus aureus* (MRSA) and staphylococcal epidermis are major pathogens. Many believe this is due to previous overuse of cephalosporins.

- We are unable to predict the consequences of antibiotic use on resistance patterns. The evolution of the prominent role of enterococci should perhaps have been predictable on the basis of early observations of superinfections during cephalosporin use. Vancomycin-resistant enterococci may reflect the use of vancomycin for staphylococci.

The consistent message from 50 years of antibiotic use is that extensive use of these drugs, no matter how well justified, *will* result in bacterial resistance, i.e. we should not use SDD even if it *were* effective in reducing the incidence of organ failures or mortality. Stomach acid is a an important protector from GI bacterial overgrowth. Thus avoiding drugs such as ranitidine that impair stomach acid secretion may offer some protection.

Prevention of stress ulceration

- Some degree of 'stress erosion or ulceration' is common in 70–100% of ICU patients on gastroscopy. These stress ulcers appear almost immediately with critical illness.

- Clinically significant ulceration, i.e. causing significant bleeding, is less common (5%)[9] and life-threatening haemorrhage is rare.

- The incidence is probably reduced in recent years due to improved and earlier resuscitation-preventing gastric mucosal ischaemic damage.[9]

- However, an unexplained drop in haemoglobin (Hb) should always make one suspect occult GI bleeding in patients at risk from stress ulcers.

- The problem is due to mucosal ischaemia not hyperacidity. Thus the logical approach for treatment is to improve mucosal protection and, indeed, the first priority is adequate resuscitation and improvement of oxygen transport to the gastric mucosa.

Patients most at risk include:

- head injuries;

- major burns;

- sepsis;

- prolonged IPPV;

- multiple trauma;

- coagulopathy;

- history of peptic ulcer.

Prophylaxis

- Antacids and H_2-blockers, such as ranitidine, are the traditional therapies for stress ulcers and are effective in reducing the incidence of bleeding.

- It has been suggested that when using antacids or H_2-blockers, gastric pH should be monitored and maintained pH >4.

- Enteral nutrition is also probably effective at preventing ulceration.

- Sucralfate may be as effective as H_2-blockers at preventing bleeding and may be associated with a reduced mortality rate.[6]

Sucralfate

- Sucralfate (sucrose aluminium sulphate) is a non-absorbable agent that protects the gastric mucosa by:

- adsorbing pepsin and bile salts;

- increasing prostaglandin secretion;

- promoting epithelial healing;

- stimulating mucous secretion;

- increasing mucosal blood flow;

- increasing bicarbonate secretion.

It has a weak bacterial inhibitory effect *in vitro*.

- Concern has been raised about the role of organisms from the GI tract in nosocomial pneumonia. Normally, the acid pH in the stomach suppresses bacterial growth. Antacids and ranitidine raise gastric pH and allow colonization of the stomach by organisms from the mouth and the rest of the GI tract. These organisms may be a source of infection.

- Studies have now shown a reduced incidence of pneumonia in patients receiving prophylaxis with sucralfate.[10] Sucralfate is cheap and virtually free of side effects. It usefully combines stress ulcer protection and possibly reduced nosocomial pneumonias with the benefit of maintained stomach acid secretion.

- 1 G (5 ml suspension) 6 hourly or 2 G 8 hourly is either swallowed or more commonly administered down a nasogastric tube. The tube should be flushed with H_2O to ensure delivery into the stomach.

Hepatic dysfunction in ICU

Acute and chronic liver failure are out of the scope of this text. These conditions are primarily 'medical' and few patients are admitted to general ICUs. Two main syndromes of hepatic dysfunction occur in ICU patients.[11] Both are relatively common and the occurrence and degree of dysfunction have adverse prognostic significance.

- *Ischaemic hepatitis*. Due to reduced hepatic perfusion during shock. Causes necrosis with, often massive, elevations of AST within 24 h. Coagulopathy, hypoglycaemia and increased lactate (partly due to reduced hepatic clearance) are often seen. May predispose to the commoner:

- *ICU jaundice*. More gradual onset (the liver has considerable reserve). Associated with sepsis (should prompt search for occult sepsis), trauma and massive blood transfusion and is the liver component of multiple organ failure. Intrahepatic cholestasis produces marked hyperbilirubinaemia with only mild elevation of enzymes.

In both situations, Kupffer cell (hepatic macrophage) dysfunction may predispose to bacterial or endotoxin translocation from the gut, exacerbating the hepatic dysfunction and promoting further general organ dysfunction.

Therapeutic principles include maintaining overall cardiac output, actively increasing liver blood flow with, e.g. dopexamine, eradication of sepsis and early enteral feeding.

Gastrointestinal disease as a cause of admission to ICU

Pancreatitis

The mortality rate is 5–10%. The rate of the more severe form, acute necrotizing pancreatitis, is 25–45%.

Aetiology

- Alcohol and gallstones account for ~80%.

- Other causes include:

    - abdominal trauma;

    - post-abdominal surgery and post-ERCP;

    - drug induced;

    - metabolic, e.g. hypercalcaemia and hyper triglycerideaemia;

    - infections, e.g. mumps and viral hepatitis

- 10% idiopathic – possibly associated with biliary sludge.

Pathogenesis

- Incompletely understood.

- Pancreastasis is probably the underlying cause leading to a reversal of the normal secretary pathways resulting in increased blood levels of enzymes.

- The reversal of the secretary pathways causes an oxidative stress[12] with increased O_2 free-radical activity. There is also a decrease in the body's antioxidant defences.

- The increase in enzyme activity leads to 'autodigestion' of pancreatic tissue, SIRS similar to sepsis, interstitial pancreatic oedema and necrosis/oedema of peripancreatic tissue.

- Severe cases cause necrosis of part of the gland and surrounding fatty tissue with haemorrhage.

Clinical presentation

- Pain – radiating to the back in 50%.

- No rebound tenderness (pancreas is retroperitoneal).

- Nausea and vomiting.

- Low grade fever.

- Abdominal distension (fluid sequestration plus ileus).

- Increase in blood enzyme levels (amylase only 70% specific. Lipase more specific with urinary trypsinogen promising).

Imaging

- Ultrasound often of limited use.

- CT of prime importance to stage and define the illness and for therapeutic interventiona and prognosis.

Management

Conventional management is supportive and includes (few subjected to controlled trials):

- 'Rest the pancreas' with nil orally and nasogatric suction.

- Analgesia.

- Intravenous fluids and nutritional support

All other interventions are arguably controversial including:

- 'Resting the pancreas' disputed by some.

- Controversy over prophylactic antibiotics with some reports of benefit.[13]

- Peritoneal lavage probably not helpful.

- Drugs, e.g. Aprotinin, glucagon, steroids of no convincing benefit. Octreotide (a somatostatin analogue) shows promise.[14]

- ERCP may be indicated in recurrent pancreatitis to ensure biliary drainage.

- Haemofiltration to remove enzymes and inflammatory molecules is associated with anecdotal reports of improvements but no formal trials.

- Antioxidant therapies have their advocates, based on strong theoretical and circumstantial evidence[12] but, again, formal trials are awaited.

The role of surgery

There is a wide variation of surgical practice in acute pancreatitis. Operative intervention carries a high mortality and many surgeons reserve surgery for patients with abscess or infected necrosis. CT-guided drainage of collections and abscesses is increasingly preferred.

Complications

- Inflammatory masses are common for 1–2 weeks. Development of abscess, pseudocyst and especially necrotizing pancreatitis are significant complications.

- Other complications are similar to those of sepsis, i.e. ARDS, renal failure and other organ failures.

Prognosis

- The most widely quoted scoring system is that of Ranson on admission with points awarded for factors such as age, WCC, glucose, liver enzymes, urea, calcium, fluid sequestration, etc. with higher points associated with a worse prognosis.

- Recent studies have focused on APACHE II scores or systemic effects, e.g. respiratory failure, requirement for inotropic support, secondary sepsis and renal insufficiency.

- CT scoring systems as indicators of prognosis have been developed[15] based on peripancreatic inflammation or collections plus degree of necrosis.

Upper gastrointestinal bleeding

GI bleeding is a common cause of admission to hospital but the majority do not require admission to ICU. This is, in part, due to the differences between traumatic shock (tissue injury) and haemorrhagic shock (GI bleed) as described in the chapter on multiple injury. Most respond well to *prompt* resuscitation. However, the overall mortality is probably unchanged at approximately 14%, mainly in the elderly, for the last 20–30 years. An increase in incidence in the elderly is probably responsible for this apparent lack of therapeutic progress.

Reasons for admission to ICU include:

- aspiration of blood;

- prolonged surgery (see chapter on the surgical patient);

- massive blood transfusion with its risk of hypothermia, coagulopathy and ARDS;

- persistent shock.

Cause of bleeding

- Peptic ulcer ~50%

- Gastric erosion ~25%

- Varices ~10%

- Others ~20%

Note: beware a history of aortic surgery.

Management

- Resuscitation along principles described in this text.

- Specialist, multidisciplinary teams including *early* surgical referral.

- Early endoscopy – important prognostic and diagnostic information.

- Endoscopic therapy – endoscopic intervention has revolutionized management of upper GI bleed and reduced the need for surgery. Ulcers can be injected around and into vessels with adrenaline, sclerosing agents or fibrin. However, 15–20% will rebleed. Risk factors have been identified and include:

  - large initial bleed;

  - shock;

  - large transfusion;

  - bleed in inpatients;

  - severe coexisting disease;

  - coagulopathy;

  - old age.

- Early surgery for endoscopic failure.

- Ongoing management of peptic ulceration.

Oesophageal varices

- Mortality is high because of the associated liver dysfunction and portal hypertension.

- The role of vasopressors to reduce bleeding is uncertain. Octreotide is possibly of no use, somatostatin uncertain and glypressin may be better.

- Sengstaken tubes to tamponade the bleeding are useful if the patient is exsanguinating but placement is difficult.

- Better endoscopic management of varices is probably reducing the incidence of bleeding.

Lower gastrointestinal bleeding

Approximately 20% of all acute GI bleeding. Commonly due to:

- diverticular disease;

- angiodysplasia;

- colonic carcinoma;

- inflammatory bowel disease.

Upper GI sources of bleeding must be excluded, followed by colonoscopy and/or angiography. Surgery is usually required and may be the reason for admission to ICU.

Other conditions

Patients with other conditions, (e.g. faecal peritonitis or severe colitis) may require admission to ICU because of prolonged surgery or septic shock.

Further Reading

Mythen MG, Webb AR. The role of gut mucosal hypoperfusion in the pathogenesis of post-operative organ dysfunction. *Int Care Med* 1994; **20**: 203–9.

Swank GM, Deitch EA. Role of the gut in multiple organ failure: bacterial translocation and permeability changes. *World J Surg* 1996; **20**: 411–17.

Grace PA. Ischaemia-reperfusion injury. *Br J Surg* 1994; **81**: 637–47.

Tryba M. Stress ulcer prophylaxis – quo vadis? *Int Care Med* 1994: **20**: 311–13.

Mergener K, Baillie J. Acute pancreatitis. *BMJ* 1998: **316**: 44–8.

Kankaria AG, Fleischer DE. The critical care management of nonvariceal upper gastrointestinal bleeding. *Crit Care Clin* 1995: **11**: 347–68.

References

1. Peitzman AB, Udekwu AO, Ochoa J, Smith S. Bacterial translocation in trauma patients. *J Trauma* 1991; **31**: 1083–6.

2. Mythen MG, Webb AR. Perioperative plasma volume expansion reduces the incidence of gut mucosal hypoperfusion during cardiac surgery. *Arch Surg* 1995; **130**: 423–9.

3. Silverman HJ, Tuma P. Gastric tonometry in patients with sepsis. Effects of dobutamine infusions and packed red blood cell transfusions. *Chest* 1992; **102**: 184–8.

4. Fink MP. Adequacy of gut oxygenation in endotoxemia and sepsis. *Crit Care Med* 1993; **21(2 suppl.)**: S4–8.

5. Selective Decontamination of the Digestive Tract Trialists' Collaborative Group. Meta-analysis of randomised controlled trials of selective decontamination of the digestive tract. *BMJ* 1993; **307**: 525–32.

6. Cook DJ, Reeve BK, Guyatt GH *et al*. Stress ulcer prophylaxis in critically ill patients. Resolving discordant meta-analyses. *JAMA* 1996; **275**: 308–14.

7. Sijpkens YW, Buurke EJ, Ulrich C, van Asselt GJ. *Enterococcus faecalis* colonisation and endocarditis in five intensive care patients as late sequelae of selective decontamination. *Int Care Med* 1995; **21**: 231–4.

8. Bartlett JG. Selective decontamination of the digestive tract and its effect on antimicrobial resistance. *Crit Care Med* 1995; **23**: 613–15.

9. Zandstra DF, Stoutenbeek CP. The virtual absence of stress-ulceration related bleeding in ICU patients receiving prolonged mechanical ventilation without any prophylaxis. A prospective cohort study. *Int Care Med* 1994; **20**: 335–40.

10. Eddleston JM, Vohra A, Scott P *et al*. A comparison of the frequency of stress ulceration and secondary pneumonia in sucralfate- or ranitidine-treated intensive care unit patients. *Crit Care Med* 1991; **19**: 1491–6.

11. Hawker F. Liver dysfunction in critical illness. *Anaesth Int Care* 1991; **19**: 165–81.

12. Braganza JM, Chaloner C. Acute pancreatitis. *Curr Opin Anaesthesiol* 1995; **8**: 126–31.

13. Sainio V, Kemppainen E, Puolakkainen P *et al*. Early antibiotic treatment in acute necrotising pancreatitis. *Lancet* 1995; **346**: 663–7.

14. Fiedler F, Jauernig G, Keim V *et al*. Octreotide treatment in patients with necrotizing pancreatitis and pulmonary failure. *Int Care Med* 1996; **22**: 909–15.

15. Patel AG, Horn EM, Karetsky M. Acute pancreatitis: current concepts of risk stratification and management. *Int Care World* 1996; **13**: 164–7.

19

THE COMATOSE PATIENT

This chapter will concentrate on the commonest causes of coma in the ICU – head injury and 'stroke' (cerebral infarction and haemorrhage). The general principles of management of these patients are applicable for other conditions which lead to coma in the ICU. Other causes of coma and an account of other neurological conditions in the ICU can be found in Wijdicks (1996) in Further Reading.

General points

- The hallmark of diffuse brain injury is loss of consciousness. Coma is unconsciousness where patients neither open eyes, obey commands or utter recognizable words.

- The severity of the patient's condition may be gauged by the depth or duration of coma.

- Duration of coma can only be judged in retrospect so therefore the depth of coma as quantified by the Glasgow Coma Scale (GCS) is widely used as an index of the severity of injury:

Eye opening		Verbal response		Motor response	
Spontaneous	4	Oriented	5	Obeys commands	6
To voice	3	Confused speech	4	Localizes pain	5
To pain	2	Inappropriate words	3	Withdraws	4
None	1	Incomprehensible sounds	2	Abnormal flexion	3
		None	1	Extension	2
				None	1

Score 3–15
Mild head injuries 14 or 15
Moderate 9–13
Severe 8 or less.

General care of the comatose patient

- Skilled nursing care especially with regard to pressure area care and protection of joints.

- Physiotherapy – both respiratory care and prevention of contractures in immobile limbs.

- Nutrition and hydration must be maintained.

- Stress ulcer prophylaxis – head injuries are at particular risk (Cushing's ulcer).

Aims of intensive care

- Detect and treat complications of primary injury that may cause delayed damage.

- Prevent delayed hypoxic/ischaemic damage – largely through control of ICP.

- Provide optimal conditions for recovery of brain function – natural recovery only at present, perhaps therapy aided neurological recovery in the future.

Principles of neuroprotection

- Factors causing increases in intracranial pressure should be avoided.

- Encourage venous drainage and therefore minimize ICP by maintaining the neck in a neutral position. Minimize the use of PEEP and where possible nurse with head up by 10°.

- Indications, complications and management of ICP monitoring will be discussed in the section on Head Injury.

- Avoid hypotension. There is a loss of normal blood pressure (BP)/cerebral blood flow (CBF) autoregulation. Normal relationship (see figure 19.1 overleaf):

Normally CBF is constant between MAP = 50–100.

- *Autoregulation.* This relationship may be lost in, for example, head injury, i.e. the head-injury patient is predisposed to ischaemic brain damage at levels of MAP normally considered satisfactory.

- *Hyperventilation* to reduce ICP. Controversial (see below).

- *Mannitol* to reduce ICP. Mannitol 50–100 G if above ineffective. Continue until osmolarity reaches 320 mosm/l.

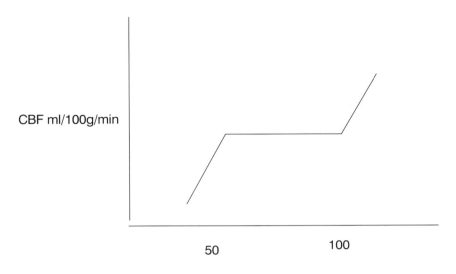

CBF ml/100g/min

50   100

Figure 19.1:   Autoregulation of cerebral blood flow

- *Hyperglycaemia.* Animal studies and studies on stroke patients clearly show increased neuronal damage after global brain ischaemia in the presence of hyperglycaemia.[1]

- *Fever* is thought to be harmful – by increasing cerebral metabolic oxygen requirements. Initial studies of head injury suggest that controlled hypothermia improves outcome.[2]

- *Steroids* have no proven role in the management of head injury or stroke.[3]

- *Indomethacin* infusion (a cerebral vascoconstrictor) reduces ICP but there may be a rebound if stopped suddenly.

- *Experimental strategies.* Interest is focusing on neuroprotective drugs (animal studies so far), e.g. free radical scavengers, inhibitors of lipid peroxidation, glutamate antagonists and calcium channel blockers.

- *Calcium antagonists* prevent calcium influx in an ischaemic area and decrease cell damage. Their smooth muscle-relaxing properties also reduce vasospasm.

- On theoretical grounds, the combination of barbiturates (to reduce cerebral oxygen demand) and positive inotropic drugs (to maintain cardiac output and MAP) is attractive but remains experimental.

The problem of hyperventilation

- CBF and therefore ICP is directly related to pCO_2 with, e.g., a fall in $pCO_2 = 1$ mmHg being normally associated with a fall in ICP of ~ 1.3 mmHg. This effect may be short lived due to brain and CSF pH compensation.

- In controlled studies *prophylactic* hyperventilation (i.e. in the absence of raised ICP) resulted in a slightly worse outcome compared with the control group.[4] The danger of hyperventilation is that it may produce excessive cerebral vasoconstriction and ischaemia.

- It seems illogical somehow to treat brain ischaemia by measures that reduce CBF. No other organ in the body is treated in this way.

- Hyperventilation will shift the haemoglobin (Hb) oxygen dissociation cure to the left impairing tissue oxygenation – regardless of any contested effect on CBF.

- An interesting study on head injury patients compared different therapies to lower ICP – 25 G i.v. mannitol, 3 min of CSF drainage via ventriculostomy and increase in respiratory rate of 4/min.[5] For similar decrease of ICP, hyperventilation caused decreases in SJO_2 (implying worsening cerebral oxygenation by reducing CBF) while mannitol increased SJO_2. CSF drainage was in between but not nearly as bad as hyperventilation.

- Thus, mannitol improved CBF while decreasing ICP and this study supports many centres avoidance of 'routine' hyperventilation.

- Although the routine use of hyperventilation is debatable there is no doubt that hypercapnia is harmful and should be avoided.

- The majority of centres still practice *therapeutic* hyperventilation for short-term control of raised ICP. Many use JVO_2 measurements as a guide. Jugular saturations $<55-60\%$ may indicate that hyperventilation is harmful.

ICP monitoring

- Although the origin of raised ICP after head injury is still debated, rational management of the injured-brain depends on knowledge of cerebral perfusion pressure (CPP), i.e. MAP – ICP.

- ICP monitoring has been widespread since the 1970s since several reports indicated a reduced mortality in severe head injuries (GCS <8) subsequent to its use. However, it is impossible to separate the contribution of ICP monitoring to this improved survival from other advances, e.g. routine CT scanning.

- Nevertheless, there is a definite association between raised ICP and poor outcome although cause and effect have never been proven. Certainly, uncontrollable increases in ICP represent overwhelming brain damage.

- Several large, non-randomized trials have shown a beneficial effect on head injury mortality from the use of ICP monitoring.[6,7]

- ICP measurement is more useful when combined with measurement of jugular venous saturations (SJO_2), which correlate inversely with CBF. With this information, therapy such as hyperventilation which can lower CBF can be more accurately judged.

Indications

- GCS <8.

- Evidence raised ICP on CT scan.

- Any CT abnormality.

- Post-craniotomy for mass lesion.

- Space occupying mass lesion.

- Traumatic coma as part of multiple trauma requiring IPPV.

Contraindications

- Frank coagulopathy.

- Obvious infection at insertion site.

- Paediatric head injury unless in specialized centres.

Complications of ICP monitoring

- Haemorrhage requiring neurosurgical intervention – perhaps 5% in some studies.

- Infection.

- Occlusion of fluid-filled monitoring systems.

Complications are low compared with other ICU interventions.

- One study[8] from Italy of ICP monitors inserted by ICU staff as opposed to neurosurgeons found the incidence of morbidity (3.3%) to be comparable with that of CVP monitoring. There were no intracranial haematomas attributed to the monitor in their 5-year study.

- Another study found that ICP monitors are safe with the main problem being accidental removal! ICP monitoring led to therapeutic changes in 81% of patients.[9]

- Older studies suggest a 10% incidence of infection. It is believed that the incidence with modern solid-state or fibreoptic systems (i.e. not fluid-based) will be considerably less (3% in reference 8). Of course the disadvantage of the modern systems is that CSF drainage for therapeutic reduction of ICP is not possible.

Control of raised ICP

The skull contains brain, blood and CSF. An increase in volume of one must be accompanied by a decrease in another or pressure will rise. Initially the volume increase be it due to haematoma or increased CBF (hyperaemia) is compensated by displacement of CSF followed by later *large* increases in ICP for a *small* further increase in volume. This may lead to:

- acute hydrocephalus due to obstruction of CSF flow;

- reduced CBF; and

- brain stem herniation at the foramen magnum ('coning').

Although the normal ICP is <10 mmHg there is general agreement that treatment is indicated when ICP >20. The mainstays of treatment are mannitol and therapeutic hyperventilation as discussed previously. Transient elevations occur during turning, physiotherapy, etc. and do not usually require treatment. A bolus of sedation in the ventilated patient may be all that is required to prevent these transient elevations in the patients most at risk, e.g. already elevated ICP. Care should be taken, however, to maintain CPP. In all cases of persistent elevation of ICP a cause should be sought, e.g. obstructed venous drainage of the head. 'Fighting' the ventilator should be excluded. When no cause is apparent repeat CT may be indicated.

Head Injury

Approximately 100,000 patients with head injuries are admitted to hospital each year in the UK of which ~10,000 are severe.

Most studies show a preponderance of males to females of between 2:1 and 4:1. The peak ages are in the second and third decades. Common causes are:

- road traffic accident (RTA);

- falls;

- assault;

- gunshot (especially in the USA).

Younger patients are commonly due to RTA – lower incidence of mass lesions on CT scanning. Older patients are commonly due to falls – higher incidence of mass lesions. Depending on aetiology, 10–50% are intoxicated on admission. 50% of multiple injury patients include a CNS component and brain injury is present in 75% of deaths from RTA.

Pathophysiology

Primary brain injury

This occurs within milliseconds and the only effective treatment is prevention. The fact that some patients who subsequently die were conscious at the scene of an accident implies that there are secondary or delayed injuries which, in theory, may be preventable or reversible.

Secondary brain injury

In most cases later secondary damage is focal, i.e. it is related to contusions and/or haematomas but may also be due to metabolic changes, raised ICP *and* extracranial events such as hypoxaemia, hypotension and hypercarbia.

CT scanning

- CT scanning remains the neuroradiologic scanning method of choice in head injuries and can evaluate skull fractures, major contusions, haematomas and cervical spine.

- It can only provide information about ICP *at the time of scanning* (may get delayed increase). Effacement of basal cisterns is usually present when ICP >20.

- In general, scanning should be delayed until oxygenation and systemic BP are satisfactory.

- Early studies suggested that only a small proportion of patients with a normal CT scan develop raised ICP. Recent studies, however,[10] suggest that severely injured patients with a normal scan are at substantial risk of developing intracranial hypertension.

- The prognosis in severe head injury is best when haematomas are diagnosed by CT and evacuated prior to the patient's deterioration from subsequent rises in ICP or local mass effect. With increasing use of CT scanning, smaller mass lesions or 'smear' haematomas may be found. Serial CTs may help evaluate these patients. For patients at risk of delayed haemorrhage or oedema, repeat CTs may be necessary, e.g. at 24 and 72 h, and 7 days. Unexpected deterioration (clinically or persist-ent rises ICP) should prompt a repeat scan to exclude the development of secondary hydrocephalus or intracranial bleeding.

Management

As for all trauma patients, *ABC* and *VIP* principles are crucial. If these are not maintained appropriately the neurologic outcome is likely to be poor because of secondary ischaemic/hypoxic brain damage – even if the patient 'survives'.

General management

*A*irway must be maintained. Neck should be immobilized in a cervical collar due to association of head injury with C spine injury until C spine shown to be intact.

*B*reathing. Indications for intubation include:

- loss of protective laryngeal reflexes;

- GCS <8;

- severe facial and/or multiple injuries;

- hypercapnia, hypoxaemia or marked tachypnoea;

- preparation for transfer;

- presence of seizures.

*C*irculation. Head injury in the absence of other injuries is almost never associated with hypotension. Normal MAP should be maintained or even supranormal MAP if ICP is raised (see below).

*V*entilation. 20% may be hypoxic without chest injury.

- Neurogenic pulmonary oedema.

- Aspiration.

- V/Q mismatch.

- Pulmonary emboli include fat emboli after long bone fractures.

- Nosocomial pneumonia (high incidence).

Appropriate respiratory care will maintain appropriate oxygenation. PEEP should be avoided or at least minimized where possible as it can restrict cerebral venous drainage and therefore contribute to raised ICP.

Duration of ventilatory support is controversial in head injured patients.

- If ICP monitoring is employed, IPPV is continued until ICP is stable and has settled to near normal. Increasing ICP during weaning leads to resedation.

- If no ICP monitoring, many now suggest a minimum period of sedation and ventilation of 3 days to allow the oedema to settle. Some centres repeat the CT scan prior to allowing the patient to awaken.

Infusion. Appropriate fluids should be administered. The presence of other injuries will necessitate appropriate volume resuscitation. Fluid infusion will not necessarily increase ICP.[11] Volume infusion is therefore 'safe'. Dextrose containing fluids should probably be avoided.

Perfusion. CPP must be maintained especially in the presence of raised ICP (CPP = MAP –ICP). Increasing emphasis in the literature is being placed on maintaining CPP at >70. It would also seem as if maintaining CPP by increasing MAP is almost to be preferred to maintaining CPP by lowering ICP – especially if ICP is resistant to therapy.[12]

Additional measures include:

- attention to the principle of neuroprotection (see above);

- nasogastric tube for gastric decompression (gastric atony common); and for early enteral nutrition – patients with head injury can be markedly catabolic;

- stress ulcer prophylaxis;

- physiotherapy;

- antibiotics prophylactically if ICP monitored. Prophylactic antibiotics are not indicated otherwise in head injury;[13]

- routine anticonvulsants, e.g. phenytoin is recommended by some authorities;

- nimodipine if traumatic subarachnoid injury present – to reduce associated vasospasm.

Outcome and quality control

The mortality from severe head injuries is 30–50% in most series. Factors suggesting a poor outcome include:

- low GCS;

- increased age;

- significant haemorrhage;

- significant systemic injuries.

50% who die do so from uncontrolled increases in ICP (often early).

A small number of patients will be left in a persistent vegetative state or alert but totally dependent. The numbers of these are *not* increased in studies involving aggressive management strategies shown to reduce mortality. Recovery may continue for up to 24 months but most improvement occurs in first 6 months.

In a study of 41 US trauma centres[14] the outcomes varied from 43% below expected to 52% above expected. 70% of this variation in outcome was found in patients with *moderate* head injuries rather than severe. The outcomes varied enormously between different centres. The implication is that the quality of prehospital and ICU care can be expected to have a profound effect on the outcome after head injury.

Stroke

Subarachnoid haemorrhage

- Studies vary but ~10–30 per 100,000 per year incidence (i.e. 10% of all cerebrovascular accidents (CVAs)).

- Aneurysms identified in 75–80% but no discrete bleeding source found in 15–20%.

- Hypertension is a significant risk factor for the development and for rupture of aneurysms.

- Peak age is 55–60 years.

- Females more than males.

Pathophysiology of rupture

The resulting increase in ICP reduces CBF and is responsible for the decrease in conscious level in all but the mildest cases. This increase in ICP may help stop the bleeding by a 'tamponade' effect! Initial non-survivors and those patients admitted in a deep, persistent coma develop persistent increases in ICP, secondary vasospasm and cerebral oedema.

There is a surge in catecholamine levels which can cause:

- myocardial ischaemia;

- arrhythmias;

- tachycardias;

- prolonged QT interval on the electrocardiogram (ECG) (itself associated with ventricular arrhythmias);

- decreases in serum K (due to the action of adrenaline on the β2 receptor).

Clinical presentation
- Headache in 85–95%.

- Nausea and vomiting.

- Decreased conscious level.

- Photophobia.

- Variety of neurological deficits.

Diagnosis
- *CT scan*. Mainstay of diagnosis and gives information on location of bleed and likely origin. May also indicate the likelihood of development of vasospasm, e.g. in the presence of significant amounts of blood in the basal cisterns.

- *MRI scan*. Although not the initial investigation of choice, this may show even very small aneurysms.

- *Lumbar puncture(LP)*. Very sensitive especially the presence of xanthochromia (yellow discolouration of the CSF due to the presence of altered blood). A CT scan should be done first to detect increased ICP as performing an LP in a patient with increased ICP can cause brain herniation.

- *Angiography*. Needed to define the source of bleeding (and the presence of other aneurysms) to guide surgery.

Non-operative management
- Non-operative management is associated with a high mortality rate.

- Attention to the principles of neuroprotection (see above).

- Surgical referral is indicated in all patients apart from those in persistent coma.

- Rebleeding occurs in 16–25% of patients in the first 2 weeks with a peak incidence at 4–9 days.[15]

- If surgery is not feasible, measures should be taken to try and lessen the risk of rebleeding, e.g. control hypertension, and treat constipation to prevent straining and vasospasm. The use of antifibrinolytics to reduce rebleeding worsens mortality.[16]

Prevention and treatment of vasospasm

The two mainstays of treatment to prevent vasospasm are:

- Nimodipine. Given i.v. as soon as possible at 1–2 mg/h (less if BP unstable) and continued for 5–14 days, followed by oral nimodipine, 60 mg 4 hourly. Hypertension must be avoided. This therapy has been clearly shown to improve outcome.[17]

- Hypervolaemic hypertensive therapy, i.e. generous fluid therapy and/or vasopressors to maintain a high BP, will reduce the incidence of vasospasm.[18] This must only be practised following surgical intervention.

- Nevertheless, before or after surgery, hypotension and hypovolaemia should be avoided.

Surgical intervention

The timing of surgical intervention has always been controversial. In the 1960s surgery was delayed and outcome was often poor. In the 1970s and 1980s early surgery was claimed to offer better results. It seems that there are similar results for surgery at 0–3 and 11–14 days. The worst outcome seems to be for surgery between days 7 and 10 due to the development of vasospasm. In other words, early or late surgery but not in between.[19]

Intravenous nimodipine should be continued for 5 days postoperatively.

Prognosis

One-third of patients will die before reaching medical attention. Of the remaining about one-third will die or remain severely disabled. An international cooperative study found that 58% returned to their premorbid state.[20]

Cerebral infarction

Ischaemic stroke is a common cause of coma in patients admitted to many ICUs. However, the role of ICU is controversial. On the one hand, prognosis is undoubtedly poor following a major cerebral ischaemic event:

- Realistically, IPPV in the absence of definitive therapy able to restore brain function cannot be expected to improve survival.

- A retrospective review of almost 1000 patients concluded that IPPV only delays an inevitable fatal outcome in patients with respiratory failure following ischaemic stroke.[21]

- Another study suggests discontinuing IPPV for patients who remain comatose for >72 h following stroke.[22]

On the other hand, some centres dispute this nihilistic attitude:

- 'Stoke units' for ' brain attack' (analogous to coronary care units for heart attack) result in reduced mortality and complications for stroke patients compared to medical wards.[23] However, this may be due, in part, to better rehabilitation rather than better acute care.

- Despite some increased incidence of intracranial haemorrhage, treatment with recombinant tissue plasminogen activator within 3 hr of the onset of an ischaemic stroke improves outcome.[24] Intravenous streptokinase causes an unacceptable incidence of haemorrhage.

- The challenge (beyond the reach of most units) is to diagnose infarction (i.e. rule out haemorrhage) within 3 hr by CT scanning to identify those who are candidates for thrombolysis.

- Surgical decompression to reduce ICP is being investigated for patients with massive hemispheric infarction with initial encouraging results.[25]

Management

- Attention to the principle of neuroprotection (see above).

- Treat severe hypertension but take care not to produce ischaemia from hypotension.

- ICP monitoring is of limited value in massive stroke.

- Look for sources of emboli, e.g. ECHO to look for valve lesions or intracardiac thrombi, auscultate carotid arteries for bruits. Consider antiplatelet drugs or anticoagulants if emboli likely.

- Nimodopine orally may have a slight protective effect when given within 12 hr but the results are not as impressive as for SAH. Intravenous nimodopine causes too much hypotension and should not be given.

Further Reading

Wijdicks EF. Neurologic complications in critically ill patients. *Anesth Analg* 1996; **83**: 411–19.

Gentleman D, Dearden M, Midgley S, Maclean D. Guidelines for resuscitation and transfer of patients with serious head injury. *BMJ* 1993; **307**: 547–52

Diringer MN. Intracerebral hemorrhage: pathophysiology and management. *Crit Care Med* 1993; **21**: 1591–603.

Hacke W, Stingele R, Steiner T *et al*. Critical care of acute ischemic stroke. *Int Care Med* 1996; **21**: 856–62.

References

1. Weir CJ, Murray GD, Dyker AG, Lees KR. Is hyperglycaemia an independent predictor of poor outcome after acute stroke? Results of a long term follow up study. *BMJ* 1997; **314**: 1303–6.

2. Marion DW, Obrist WD, Carlier PM *et al*. The use of moderate therapeutic hypothermia for patients with severe head injuries: a preliminary report. *J Neurosurg* 1993; **79**: 354–62

3. Alderson P, Roberts I. Corticosteroids in acute traumatic brain injury: a systematic review of randomised controlled trials. *BMJ* 1997; **314**: 1855–9.

4. Muizelaar JP, Marmarou A, Ward JD *et al*. Adverse effects of prolonged hyperventilation in patients with severe head injury: a randomized clinical trial. *J Neurosurg* 1991; **75**: 731–9.

5. Fortune JB, Feustel PJ, Graca L *et al*. Effect of hyperventilation, mannitol and ventriculostomy drainage on cerebral blood flow after head injury. *J Trauma* 1995; **39**: 1091–9.

6. Miller JD, Becker DP, Ward JD. Significance of intracranial hypertension in severe head injury. *J Neurosurg* 1977; **47**: 503–16.

7. Marshall LF, Smith RW, Shapiro HM. The outcome with aggressive treatment in severe head injury. Part 1. The significance of intracranial pressure monitoring. *J Neurosurg* 1979; **50**: 20–5.

8. Bochicchio M, Latronico N, Zappa S *et al*. Bedside burr hole for intracranial pressure monitoring by intensive care physicians. A 5-year experience. *Int Care Med* 1996; **22**: 1070–4.

9. Eddy VA, Vitsky JL, Rutherford EJ, Morris JA Jr. Aggressive use of ICP monitoring is safe and alters patient care. *Am J Surg* 1995; **61**: 24–9.

10. O'Sullivan MG, Statham PF, Jones PA *et al*. Role of intracranial pressure monitoring in severely head-injured patients without signs of intracranial hypertension on initial computerized tomography. *J Neurosurg* 1994; **80**: 46–50.

11. Schmoker JD, Shackford SR, Wald SL, Pietropaoli JA. An analysis of the relationship between fluid and sodium administration and intracranial pressure after head injury. *J Trauma* 1992; **33**: 476–81.

12. Andrews PJD. What is the optimal perfusion pressure after brain injury? – a review of the evidence with an emphasis on arterial pressure. *Acta Anaesthesiol Scand* 1995; **39 (suppl. 105)**: 112–14.

13. Antimicrobial prophylaxis in neurosurgery and after head injury. Infection in Neurosurgery Working Party of the British Society for Antimicrobial Chemotherapy. *Lancet* 1994; **344**: 1547–51.

14. Klauber MR, Marshall LF, Luerssen JG. Determinants of head injury mortality: importance of the low risk patient. *Neurosurgery* 1984; **24**: 3.

15. Rosenorn J, Eskesen V, Schmidt K, Ronde F. The risk of rebleeding from ruptured intracranial aneurysms. *J Neurosurg* 1987; **67**: 329–32.

16. Fodstad H, Forsell A, Liliequist B. Antifibrinolysis with tranexamic acid in aneurysmal subarachnoid haemorrhage: a consecutive controlled trial. *Neurosurgery* 1981; **28**: 21–3.

17. Allen GS, Ahn HS, Preziosi TJ. Cerebral artery spasm – a controlled trial of nimodipine in patients with subarachnoid haemorrhage. *N Engl J Med* 1983; **308**: 619–24.

18. Kassell NF, Peerless SJ, Durward QJ *et al.* Treatment of ischemic deficits from vasospasm with intravascular volume expansion and induced arterial hypertension. *Neurosurgery* 1982; **11**: 337–41.

19. Guy J, McGrath BJ, Borel CO *et al.* Perioperative management of aneurysmal subarachnoid hemorrhage: Part 1. Operative management. *Anaesth Analg* 1995; **81**: 1060–72.

20. Kassell NF, Torner JC, Haley C. The international cooperative study on the timing of aneurysmal surgery: Part 1. overall management results. *J Neurosurg* 1990; **73**: 18–32.

21. El-Ad B, Bornstein N, Fuchs P, Korczyn AD. Mechanical ventilation in stroke patients: is it worthwhile? *Neurology* 1996; **47**: 657–9.

22. Grota J, Pasteur W, Khwaja G *et al.* Elective intubation for neurological deterioration after stroke. *Neurology* 1995; **45**: 640–4.

23. Langhorne P, Williams BO, Gilchrist W, Howie K. Do stroke units save lives? *Lancet* 1993; **342**: 395–8.

24. The National Institute of Neurological Disorders and Stroke rt-PA Stroke Study Group. Tissue plasminogen activator for acute ischemic stroke. *N Engl J Med* 1995; **333**: 1581–7.

25. Rieke K, Schwab S, Krieger D *et al.* Decompressive surgery in space-occupying hemispheric infarction: results of an open, prospective trial. *Crit Care Med* 1995; **23**: 1576–87.

20

THE CRITICALLY ILL ASTHMATIC

S.G. Brear

- Acute severe asthma should be considered the unstable angina of respiratory medicine.

- Asthma kills!

Incidence

In many countries in the 30 years up to the early 1990s there was a steep rise in hospital admissions for asthma, accounting for ~100,000 per year in England and Wales, half of which are <15 years of age. In children, males have a higher admission rate than females, the opposite being true for adults. In the UK there has been a similar but less marked increase in asthma deaths, which seems to have recently levelled out.

Causes

Asthma is an inflammatory disease of the lower airways that may be associated with specific identifiable allergy (atopic or extrinsic asthma) or not (non-atopic or intrinsic asthma). The latter starts more commonly in mid and late adult life.
It is a disease of exacerbation with either full remission or persistence of symptoms (chronic severe asthma). Exacerbation may be due to:

- specific allergen exposure – environmental, food or occupational;

- air pollution – gaseous or particulate;

- treatment non-compliance;

- infection – viral or bacterial;

- thunderstorms.

Many exacerbations have no identifiable cause.

Differential diagnosis

The diagnosis may be obvious but in adults, especially in the absence of a previous history of asthma, the following alternatives should be considered:

- chronic obstructive airways disease;
- left ventricular failure;
- upper airway obstruction;
- pulmonary embolus.

Medical management

The following broadly follows the British Thoracic Society guidelines[1] on acute asthma management.

Prevention of exacerbations

Avoiding severe exacerbations is preferable by:

- avoidance of allergens;
- monitoring of peak flows and early recognition;
- avoid reliance on just bronchodilators;
- prophylactic anti-inflammatory treatment (inhaled steroids, etc.);
- longer acting β-agonists (e.g. salmeterol);
- prompt treatment of worsening symptoms (e.g. oral steroids, hospitalization);
- prompt treatment of bacterial infections when appropriate.

Presentation and signs of severity

Asthmatics may die before admission to hospital or ICU because of one or more of the following:[2]

- doctors failing to assess severity by objective measurement;
- patients and their relatives underestimating the severity of attacks;
- under treatment of attacks (e.g. under use of oral corticosteroids);
- very rapid progression from uncontrolled to life-threatening asthma.

Many clinical signs of acute severe and life-threatening asthma are unreliable. The following are the most reliable:

Acute severe asthma

- Peak expiratory flow (PEF) rate is 33–50% of predicted or best previous recorded.

- Unable to complete a sentence in one breath.

- Tachycardia >110 beats/min.

- Respiratory rate >25 breaths/min.

Life-threatening asthma

- Peak flow rate <33% of predicted or best previous recorded.

- Exhaustion, confusion, depressed level of consciousness or coma.

- Shock or bradycardia.

- Silent chest, cyanosis or feeble respiratory effort.

Not all patients with acute severe or life-threatening asthma display all features. Extreme caution should be exercised in the presence of *any* of them.

The importance of blood gas estimation

Physical signs can be unreliable. A PEF rate >33% predicted is rarely associated with CO_2 retention. All patients with oxygen saturation <92% or who have life-threatening features should have arterial blood gases measured. The following indicate a very severe attack:

- acidosis respiratory or metabolic;

- severe hypoxia (PaO_2 <8 kPa, 60 mmHg);

- normal or raised $PaCO_2$.

Initial treatment

The following measures should be taken immediately:

- oxygen in high concentration. CO_2 retention is *not* aggravated by high concentration oxygen in asthmatics;

- high-dose nebulized β_2-agonists;

- intravenous hydrocortisone 200 mg.

The patient should receive no sedatives and should have a chest X-ray to exclude pneumothorax. Response to treatment must be monitored with PEF rates and repeat blood gas estimation. If life-threatening features are present include:

- ipratropium 0.5 mg in addition to the β-agonist;
- aminophylline 250 mg i.v. over 20 min – not to be given if already on oral theophylline. Alternatively 250 μg salbutamol or terbutiline i.v.

If the patient improves with the above:

- continue a high concentration oxygen;
- give oral prednisolone 30–60 mg daily or hydrocortisone 200 mg 6 hourly;
- nebulized β-agonist 6 hourly;
- monitor patient, saturations, blood gases and PEF rates *closely*.

If the patient does not improve in 15–30 min:

- continue oxygen and steroids as above;
- give β-agonists more frequently (up to 15–30 min);
- add ipratropium 0.5 mg 6 hourly;
- consider aminophylline infusion 750–1500 mg/24 hr – dose depending on size;
- consider salbutamol or terbutiline infusion as an alternative to aminophylline.

Response to treatment must be monitored with PEF, patient 'clinical' assessment and blood gas estimations if life-threatening features persist or oximetry is <92%.

Indications for admission to ICU

Intensive care admission is indicated if:

- the PEF rate deteriorates despite treatment;
- hypoxia persists or worsens;
- hypercarbia or acidosis persists or worsens;
- the patient has impaired consciousness or exhaustion;
- respiratory effort deteriorates clinically;
- the patient is comatosed or has a respiratory arrest.

Staff able to intubate reliably must be immediately available.

Indications for intubation

Absolute indications for intubation and mechanical ventilation include:

- coma;
- respiratory arrest or ineffectual respirations;
- exhaustion.

Other considerations for early intubation include:

- progressive hypoxaemia despite increasing inspired oxygen;
- progressive hypercapnia (note that a normal $PaCO_2$ may denote a rising level passing through the normal range);
- progressive acidosis particularly if metabolic;
- ineffectual cough/retained secretions.

These non-mandatory indications should be used in conjunction with the general state and appearance of the patient.

The most experienced intubator must carry out intubation. A standard, rapid sequence method with pre-oxygenation should be used and gastric aspiration prevented using cricoid pressure. The fibreoptic bronchoscopes in ICU use will usually only fit down an ET tube >7.5 mm.

Mechanical ventilation of the asthmatic patient

Two broad, overlapping groups of patients requiring mechanical ventilation, are recognized:

Acute asphyxic asthma[3]

Characterized by:

- often short onset of action from relatively normal respiratory function baseline;
- extremely severe airflow obstruction overwhelming relatively normal respiratory muscles;
- response to treatment may be rapid but often not;
- very difficult to ventilate using standard parameters[4] – which often causes:
  - cardiovascular instability;
  - high airway pressures;

- severe air trapping with intrinsic PEEP;

- high risk of barotrauma;

- mortality from obstructive shock, tissue hypoxia or pneumothorax.

Acute severe asthma

Characterized by:

- lengthier onset of attack – may be days;

- often not from normal respiratory function baseline;

- more secretions and airway oedema problems;

- moderate or severe airway obstruction but respiratory muscle fatigue may be a greater problem;

- response of airway disease to treatment may be very slow – steroids can take many days to work;

- may be relatively easy to ventilate with standard settings;

- if respiratory muscle fatigue is the major problem then rapid recovery occurs.

Cardiovascular instability and barotrauma can be avoided by limiting peak and mean airway pressures, extending expiratory time, minimizing intrinsic PEEP, maintaining oxygen saturations >92% and supporting cardiac output.[5] This can be achieved by:

- low respiratory rates (down to 1–2/min, if necessary by manual ventilation, in extreme cases);

- low tidal volumes and low inspiratory flow rates to keep peak airway pressures <50 mmHg;

- long I:E ratios to allow adequate expiration to occur;

- high concentration oxygen to maintain adequate saturations.

This strategy will result in high concentrations of $PaCO_2$, but patients are more at risk from hypoxia, low cardiac output and barotrauma than from hypercapnia.

Pressure-controlled ventilation can be used but tidal volumes have to be monitored very closely since the fluctuating changes airway resistance typical of asthma affects tidal volume greatly.

Anecdotal therapies

There are anecdotal reports of benefit for the following treatments in very resistant asthmatic, but they should be considered after the above management fails.

Ketamine

- An i.v. anaesthetic agent that has bronchodilating properties.

- Anecdotal reports of ketamine used as an adjunct to standard bronchodilators, substituting as sedative of choice.

- Side effects include hallucinations, psychosis and increase in blood pressure.

- Less likely to be respiratory depressant and the airway better maintained than with many other anaesthetic agents.

Intravenous magnesium sulphate

- Used in both adults and children.

- Reports of improvement and even avoidance of intubation and mechanical ventilation.

- Optimal dose is unclear but as a guide, 8–16 mmol over 30–60 min followed by 64 mmol over 24 hr is a regimen suggested for arrhythmias/myocardial infarction.

Volatile anaesthetic agents

- Halothane and enflurane are the most commonly used in patients who are already intubated and ventilated.

- They have some bronchodilator effects but may be associated with cardiovascular side effects, and halothane may cause hepatotoxicity with repeated use.

- Ethyl ether has been used but is more difficult to administer.

Heliox

- Use of heliox in asthma is controversial.

- Available as a 60–80% mixture with oxygen.

- Less dense than air and offers less resistance to gas flow by encouraging laminar flow rather than turbulent flow in medium and larger airways.

- Work of breathing may be reduced and the onset of respiratory muscle fatigue delayed in awake patients.

Bronchoscopy and bronchial lavage

- Bronchoscopy can be helpful in removing the mucous plugs that may cause bronchial occlusion (particularly in the upper lobes) and worsen gas exchange.

- A tenacious nature can make secretions difficult to aspirate through the small channel of a fibreoptic bronchoscope – saline (not water) instillation can help and the procedure may need repeating.

- Single, whole-lung saline lavage has been used although it may be associated with an increase incidence of pneumonia.

Extra-corporeal membrane oxygenation (ECMO)

- ECMO has been used is some patients with success, although it has its problems.

- It is associated with a high incidence of a serious side effect, e.g. bleeding.

- It is only available in specialist centres.

- It is only considered as last resort in centres where the technique is available.

Cardiorespiratory arrest in asthmatics

Little has been written of the management of cardiorespiratory arrest in the asthmatic patient. The following applies:

- They are often unsuccessful or associated with residual cerebral anoxic damage.

- Standard resuscitation guidelines do not address the specific problems of cardiorespiratory arrest due to acute severe asthma.

- Inappropriate application of standard guidelines may turn a respiratory arrest into a cardiorespiratory arrest and death.

- Cardiac arrest may be secondary to hypoxia, electrolyte disturbance or obstructive shock.

- Often EMD or asystole.

The resuscitation recommendation of 12 breaths/min with 3–4 s for exhalation is inappropriate in intubated asthmatics following respiratory arrest, whose passive exhalation time is measured in minutes. The following problems arise:

- high levels of intrinsic PEEP;

- marked air trapping and increases in residual capacity;

- high intrathoracic pressures;

- obstructive shock with progressive reduction in cardiac output leading to cardiac arrest and cerebral hypoxic damage;

- ineffectual external cardiac massage;

- high risk of tension pneumothorax and other barotrauma.

The following measures should be considered in these extreme circumstances:

- low respiratory rates of 1–4 slow manual breaths/min or:

- apnoeic oxygenation with intratracheal oxygen insufflation (as performed during brain stem testing);[6]

- manual extrathoracic compression to mimic active exhalation and reduce intrathoracic volume;

- high suspicion of tension pneumothorax – if in doubt insert bilateral chest drains (incision/blunt dissection *not* by trochar method);

- if external cardiac massage ineffective in producing output – early recourse to internal cardiac massage.

Asthmatics *can* survive cardiorespiratory arrest but the longer the above methods are inappropriately delayed, the more likely cerebral anoxic damage will result. Patients die of a lack of cardiac output and tissue hypoxia, not of hypercapnia from hypoventilation.

Prognosis and causes of mortality

- In England and Wales there are ~2000 deaths per year in adults from asthma.

- Despite recent fears of deaths related to over treatment, most asthmatic deaths are associated with under treatment.

- Many deaths may be preventable with early recognition of exacerbation and prompt treatment particularly with systemic steroids.

- Mortality rates vary greatly in a reported series of mechanically ventilated asthmatics – from 28 to 0% – is it explained by different types/severity and the threshold for intubation between units?

- The commonest causes of death are asphyxia, cardiovascular insufficiency, cerebral hypoxia, pneumothorax and overwhelming infection.

- Many deaths occur in patients who are known to be bad asthmatics and/or who have recently been seen by a doctor for asthma.

Further reading

Levy BD, Kitch B, Fanta CH. Medical and ventilatory management of status asthmaticus. *Int Care Med* 1998; **24**: 105–17.

Cockcroft DW. Management of acute severe asthma. *Ann Aller Asthma Imm* 1995;**75**: 83–9.

References

1. The British Guidelines on Asthma Management 1995 Review and Position Statement. *Thorax* 1997; **52 (suppl. 1)**: S1.

2. Cochrane GM, Clark T. A survey of asthma mortality in patients between ages 35 and 64 in Greater London hospitals in 1971. *Thorax* 1975; **30** ; 300–5.

3. Wasserfallen JB, Schaller MD, Feihl F, Perret CH. Sudden asphyxic asthma: a distinct entity? *Am Rev Respir Dis* 1990; **142**: 108–11.

4. Tuxen DV. Detrimental effects of positive end-expiratory pressure during controlled mechanical ventilation of patients with severe airflow obstruction. *Am Rev Respir Dis* 1989; **140**; 5–9.

5. Darioli A, Perret C. Mechanical controlled hypoventilation in status asthmaticus. *Am Rev Respir Dis* 1984; **129**: 385–7.

6. Frumin MJ, Cohen G. Apnoeic oxygenation in man. *Anaesthesiology* 1959: **20**; 789–98.

21

THE CRITICALLY ILL
DIABETIC

Diabetes is a common medical condition – almost 5% of the population, although a much smaller proportion are insulin-dependent diabetics. Consideration of diabetes in this text is worthwhile not least due to the important points regarding fluid therapy in diabetic hyperglycaemic coma.

Diabetic coma, the commonest endocrine emergency, falls into three categories:

- Hypoglycaemic coma – easy to understand and treat once recognised. Therefore not discussed here.

- Diabetic ketoacidosis

- Hyperosmolar non-ketotic coma.

Diabetic ketoacidosis

Diabetic ketoacidosis (DKA) is relatively common:

- ~5% of insulin dependent diabetic patients per year;

- mainly <40 years of age, but can also affect elderly patients;

- said to affect women more than men.

- Precipitated by infection in 30%, management errors in 15% but no obvious cause in 40%. Previously undiagnosed diabetes is the cause in 10% of DKA.

The hallmarks of DKA are:

- Hyperglycaemia.

- Dehydration (5–10 litres of water) lost by osmotic diuresis, hyperventilation and vomiting.

- Loss of electrolytes – ~500 mmol in total of both sodium and potassium.

- Acidosis (ketosis and, in later stages lactic acidosis form tissue hypoperfusion).

- Much of the fluid lost, comes from the intracellular space and therefore is relatively hypotonic. Therefore, although distinction is made between DKA and Hyperosmolar non ketotic coma this is slightly arbitrary as DKA patients are always significantly hyperosmolar. Ketosis progresses to ketoacidosis when fluid loss exceeds intake due to:

  - osmotic diuresis;

  - vomiting; and

  - renal compensation overwhelmed by decreasing renal function.

Presentation

The average time of onset of condition to presentation is ~3 days. It is commonly present with combinations of the following:

Anorexia	Vomiting	Thirst
weakness	Polyuria	Weight loss
↓Conscious level	Blurred vision	Abdominal pain
GI bleed	Hyperventilation	Tachycardia
Ketones on breath	Hypotension	Hypothermia (rarely fever).

It is dangerous to assume that the abdominal pain is due to DKA. Conversely, it would be inappropriate to take a patient with DKA for laparotomy! The laboratory signs are:

- ↑blood sugar, haematocrit, urea, white blood cells (WBC), triglycerides; and

- ↓pH, bicarbonate, serum potassium, magnesium and phosphate.

The raised WBC is not necessarily an indicator of associated infection.

The interpretation of serum Na is more complex. It is well demonstrated but under appreciated that an elevated serum glucose 'dilutes' the plasma Na resulting in an inappropriately low measured Na.[1] The plasma Na decreases by ~1 mmol/l for each 3 mmol/l rise in blood sugar. In addition, if the Na is measured by a flame emission spectrophotometer technique an elevated hyperlipidaemia (as in DKA) will cause a 'pseudohyponatraemia' due to the increase of the 'solids' component of plasma. Thus a low Na may be 'normal' in DKA, a normal Na may be 'high' and a high Na signifies marked hyperosmolarity.

Indications for admission to ICU

- Most DKA patients do not need to go to ICU.
- Airway compromise.
- Severe acidosis – unless rapidly responsive to fluid therapy.
- Hypotension – unless rapidly responsive to fluid therapy.
- Hypoxia.
- Severe coexisting medical conditions.
- Lower threshold in the elderly patient.

Management

General

- The airway must be protected; by tracheal intubation if necessary.
- A nasogastric tube is essential due to the gastric atony.
- Urinary catheter – risk of renal shutdown outweighs the risk of infection.
- Close observation, regular electrolyte and blood sugar measurements.
- Infection screen but no routine antibiotics unless clinical evidence of infection.
- Subcutaneous heparin prophylaxis due to risk of thrombosis.
- CVP monitoring if hypotensive despite initial rapid fluid therapy.
- Elderly patients, severely acidotic patients, patients who do not respond to colloid infusion or patients developing ARDS (see below) warrant a PAFC.

Fluid and electrolyte therapy

Fluid replacement is the first priority taking precedence over the administration of insulin. Delay may lead to a poor outcome. Fluid therapy alone will:

- reduce the blood sugar by dilution (by up to 20%);
- restore cardiac output, organ blood flow, cardiac output and blood pressure and correct acidosis;
- restore renal function which will aid the correction of acidosis;

- deliver insulin to its tissue receptors.

The choice of fluid is controversial between 0.9% saline, 0.45% saline and colloids.

Arguments in favour of 0.9% saline being the main fluid:

- Restores plasma volume and interstitial fluid.
- Na content being higher than plasma may prevent too rapid decreases in osmolarity.
- Clinically found to be sufficient and effective for many DKA.

Arguments against large volumes of 0.9% saline:

- Danger of late hyperchloraemic acidosis.[2]
- Danger of late hypernatraemia.
- May over expand the interstitial space while not replenishing the intra-cellular space.
- Patients have lost more water than Na.

Arguments in favour of 0.45% saline:

- Closer in composition to that of fluid deficit.
- Replenishes all fluid spaces equally.
- Avoids hypernatraemia.

Arguments against 0.45% saline:

- Slow to expand plasma and interstitial spaces.
- Potentially more rapid fall in plasma osmolarity.

Arguments in favour of colloid:

- Initial rapid correction of plasma volume and shock.

Arguments against colloid:

- Not necessary for less severe cases, i.e. those not admitted to ICU.

A suggested approach is:

- Initial 1000 ml N saline rapidly if hypotensive.
- 2000 ml colloid rapidly if hypotension or acidosis are severe or no response in BP to above.
- Continue with 0.45% saline at ~500 ml/h for 4 h then ~250 ml/h so as to aim for 4–6 litres of fluid in 24 h. Be prepared to adjust according to responses.

- No 0.9% saline or colloid if Cl >110 or Na>150.

- When blood sugar <20 mmol/l switch fluids to dextrose 5% or dextrose/saline.

- Give K early in form of KCl (K phosphate if Cl high) at 20 mmol/h unless K very high (due to the acidosis) or there is no urine output. Rate may have to be increased if K very low. If K is very low Mg should also be checked.

Insulin

Soluble insulin should be given at 5–10 U/h. Previously recommended higher doses are rarely necessary.[3] The aim is to bring the blood sugar down relatively slowly over 24 hours to avoid precipitate falls in osmolarity.

Adsorption of insulin to plastic syringes is irrelevant as the infusion rate and dose are titrated to the clinical effect. Occasionally higher rates of insulin infusion are required.

Bicarbonate

Bicarbonate administration is usually unnecessary and potentially dangerous:

- Rapid falls in K as acidosis corrected.

- Shifts Hb dissociation curve to the left inhibiting tissue oxygenation.

- 8.4% Bicarbonate is extremely hyperosmolar.

- Danger of 'overshoot'.

However, a pH <7.0 may cause cardiac dysfunction. One study found no difference in outcome with bicarbonate therapy[4] and it is recommended that bicarbonate be reserved for those patients with pH <7.0 or electrocardiogram (ECG) signs of hyperkalaemia. 8.4% Na bicarbonate should be avoided or diluted in 0.45% saline. The same degree of acidosis in DKA is better tolerated than in lactic acidosis due to the lesser degree of tissue hypoxia. Interestingly the degree of acidosis does not correlate with the degree of hyperglycaemia.[5]

Phosphate

Often low. In theory replacement should replenish the low levels of 2,3-diphosphoglycerate (2,3-DPG) in red blood cells (RBC) and aid oxygen release from Hb.[6] However, the harmful effects of a low 2,3-DPG on Hb oxygen affinity are mitigated by the presence of acidosis and routine phosphate administration, with its dangers of hypocalcaemia is not recommended.

Complications of DKA

Two complications of severe DKA and therefore complications seen in DKA patients admitted to ICU are:

- *Cerebral oedema*.[7] May occur from too rapid lowering of osmolarity either by over hydration or rapid lowering of blood sugar. Is associated with an increased mortality. Unnecessary administration of bicarbonate may cause a paradoxical cerebro-spinal fluid (CSF) acidosis and cerebral oedema as carbon dioxide crosses the blood–brain barrier but bicarbonate cannot.

- *ARDS*.[8] ARDS can lead to a requirement for IPPV in severe DKA. The cause is thought to be related to severe acidosis and its effects on membrane permeability. Physiological shunt is also reported to increase despite no increase in lung water.[9]

Hypoglycaemia is a common complication of therapy of DKA.[10]

Prognosis

Reported mortality from DKA varies in the literature but in the ICU is probably ~5%. Many deaths are due to preventable metabolic complications. Increasing age and coexisting disease significantly increase mortality.[11] The mortality is probably better correlated with the osmolarity rather than the degree of acidosis. Development of either ARDS or cerebral oedema is a poor prognostic sign.

Hyperosmolar non-ketotic coma (HNC)

In HNC the abnormalities of lipid metabolism seen in DKA do not occur and therefore ketosis and acidosis is not a feature. The reason for this difference is not known for certain but one theory is that residual insulin levels may be sufficient to prevent this. Hyperglycaemia is severe, water loss is often greater – up to 25% total body water – and hyperosmolarity is marked. Most patients are >50 years of age and infection is a common precipitating cause. Mortality may approach 50%.

Hyperosmolarity *is* a feature of DKA and therefore overall presentation and management is similar with several important differences:

- Onset is slower; over 5–10 days.

- Aggressive fluid loading may lower osmolarity too rapidly, therefore slower rehydration may be appropriate. 0.45% Saline recommended.

- Often more sensitive to insulin, therefore uncommon to require more than 5 U/h.

- Empirical antibiotics are indicated due to the high incidence of associated infection.

- Thromboembolic complications are common, including hemiplegia, therefore full anticoagulation is indicated.

Further Reading

Krentz AJ, Nattrass M. Acute metabolic complications of diabetes mellitus: diabetic ketoacidosis, hyperosmolar non-ketoic syndromes and lactic acidosis. In Pickup J, Williams G (eds), *Textbook of Diabetes*, vol. 1. Oxford: Blackwells, 1997.

Hillman K. Fluid resuscitation in diabetic emergencies – a reappraisal. *Int Care Med* 1987; **13**: 4–8.

Hunt SM, Groff JL. *Advanced Nutrition and Human Metabolism*. St Paul: West, 1990.

References

1. Worthley LIG. *Handbook of Emergency Laboratory Tests*. New York: Churchill Livingstone, 1996, pp. 14–15.

2. Oh MS, Banerji MA, Carrol HJ. The mechanism of hyperchloraemic acidosis during the recovery phase of diabetic ketoacidosis. *Diabetes* 1981; **30**: 310–13.

3. Kitabachi AE. Low dose insulin therapy in diabetic ketoacidosis. Fact or fiction? *Diabetes and Metabolism Reviews* 1989; **5**: 337–41.

4. Morris LR, Murphy MB, Kitabachi AE. Bicarbonate therapy in severe diabetic ketoacidosis. *Ann Int Med* 1986; **105**: 836–40.

5. Brandt KR, Miles JM. Relationship between severity of hyperglycaemia and metabolic acidosis in diabetic ketoacidosis. *Mayo Clinic Proceedings* 1988; **63**: 1071–4.

6. Clerbaux T, Reynart M, Willems E, Frans A. Effect of phosphate on oxygen–haemoglobin affinity, diphosphoglycerate and blood gases during recovery from diabetic ketoacidosis. *Int Care Med* 1989; **1**: 495–8.

7. Hammond P, Wallis S. Cerebral oedema in diabetic ketoacidosis. *BMJ* 1992; **305**: 203–4.

8. Brun Buisson CJ, Bonnet F, Bergert S *et al*. Recurrent high permeability pulmonary oedema associated with diabetic ketoacidosis. *Crit Care Med* 1985; **13**: 55–6.

9. Laggner AN, Lenz K, Kleinberger G *et al*. Influence of fluid replacement on extravascular lung water (EVLW) in patients with diabetic ketoacidosis. *Int Care Med* 1988; **14**: 201–5.

10. Malone ML, Klos SE, Gennism VM, Goodwin JS. Frequent hypoglycaemic episodes in the treatment of patients with diabetic ketoacidosis. *Archiv Int Med* 1992; **152**: 2472–7.

11. Connell FA, Louden JM. Diabetes mortality in persons under 45 years of age. *Am J Publ Hlth* 1983; **73**: 1174–9.

INDEX